Working With Worry

A Workbook for Parents on How to Support Anxious Children

Melissa Kilbride, LICSW

Samantha Sweeney, PhD

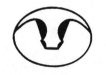

Bull Publishing Company
Boulder, Colorado

Bull Publishing Company
P.O. Box 1377
Boulder, CO USA 80306
www.bullpub.com

Library of Congress Cataloging-in-Publication Data
Names: Kilbride, Melissa, author. | Sweeney, Samantha, author.
Title: Working with worry : a workbook for parents on how to support anxious children / Melissa Kilbride, LICSW, Samantha Sweeney, PhD.
Description: 1st Edition. | Boulder : Bull Publishing Company, 2021. | Includes index. | Summary: "Working with Worry is designed to give parents practical tools they can use to support their children as they try to manage their anxiety in today's increasingly stressful world. It is a hands-on workbook that you can turn to for easy-to-understand information, recommendations, and support. Parents will learn about what anxiety looks like in children, reflect on their own experiences with anxiety, and find a wealth of intervention activities to try with their children. The activities use proven techniques including mindfulness, creativity, and self-regulation, and are organized by type of intervention, age, and areas of interest. This book is unlike any other workbook available on this subject because it offers both education and guidance around supporting children, while helping parents understand the need to be self-reflective about their own relationships with anxiety"-- Provided by publisher. Identifiers: LCCN 2020043175 (print) | LCCN 2020043176 (ebook) | ISBN 9781945188459 (paperback) | ISBN 9781945188466 (ebook)
Subjects: LCSH: Anxiety in children. | Parenting. | Parent and child.
Classification: LCC BF723.A5 .K55 2021 (print) | LCC BF723.A5 (ebook) | DDC 155.4/1246--dc23
LC record available at https://lccn.loc.gov/2020043175
LC ebook record available at https://lccn.loc.gov/2020043176

Printed in the U.S.A.

26 25 24 23 22 21   10 9 8 7 6 5 4 3 2 1

Interior design and production by Dovetail Publishing Services
Cover design and production by Shannon Bodie, Bookwise Design

Dedication

To our former and current clients,
thank you for letting us into your worlds.
For all that you've shared and taught us, we are so grateful.

To our families: Paul, Caden, and Violet; Mark, Tyler, and Lila.
Thank you for being our worlds.

About the Authors

Melissa L. Kilbride is a clinical social worker in private practice on Capitol Hill in Washington, DC. She completed her undergraduate education at the University of Michigan in Ann Arbor and received her social work degree from the Jane Addams College of Social Work at the University of Illinois–Chicago. Melissa has over fourteen years of clinical experience working with children, families, and adults. Prior to opening her own practice, she worked for the DC Department of Behavioral Health's School Mental Health Program doing individual and group counseling with children and teens, crisis intervention, and parenting workshops. Before moving to Washington, DC, Melissa was a member of the administrative team for a network of charter schools in Chicago, where she helped to create their social-emotional learning curriculum and oversaw all mental health-related services. Currently Melissa works with adults and couples with a focus on anxiety, depression, trauma, infertility, and relationship and sexual issues. She has developed "Conversation Is the New 'Talk': The Why and How of Talking to Children about Their Bodies and Sex" and other seminars for parents on topics related to early sexual health education and consent designed to help parents have conversations with more confidence.

Samantha C. Sweeney is a licensed psychologist in the District of Columbia. She has a PhD in school psychology from the University of Maryland–College Park, where she was a fellowship recipient. Samantha earned her undergraduate psychology degree from the University of Pennsylvania. Prior to opening her own practice, Samantha was a preschool teacher, a consultant and researcher in the DC public schools, and a school psychologist in the Fairfax County, Virginia, public schools. She has also worked at Wediko Children's Services Summer Program for children and adolescents with significant emotional and behavioral challenges, served as an adjunct professor in Howard University's School Psychology Program, and was a preschool screening team leader at the Kathy Wilson Foundation in Alexandria, Virginia. Samantha has a website and blog for parents to help their children develop the essential skill of cultural competence. She also speaks on the topic of cultural competence.

Acknowledgments

For your assistance and support in making this book happen, we want to thank Dr. Erica Berg, Julie Berman, Jennifer Coffey, Joan Dim, Seth Gold, Amanda Hopper, Sarah Jordan, Robin Leon, Barry Lippman, Annie McLennan, Natalie Nadler, Cynthia Serrato, Anya Stockburger, and Howard Yoon.

Thank you to our parents and siblings—Jennifer, Carol, Robert, Julie, Rene, and Barry—for their love, support, and guidance over the years. Without you, we certainly wouldn't have gotten this far and this book could not have become a reality. We love you!

A special shout-out to Christina Wiginton at Metamorphosis Book Development. Without her, this book would not have come to life the way it did.

Thank you so much to Jim Bull and the team at Bull Publishing. Your support and responsiveness has helped to quell our own anxiety as first-time authors.

Contents

Mindfulness Interventions and Exercises   99

Self-Regulation Interventions and Exercises 112

Creativity Interventions and Exercises 122

Working
With
Worry

A Workbook for Parents on
How to Support Anxious Children

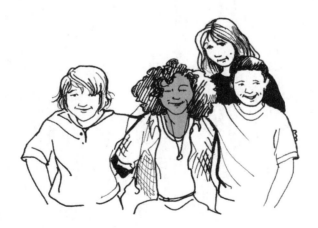

Introduction:
Welcome to Our Workbook

Welcome!

Welcome to our workbook. This book is designed to help you provide targeted and intentional support to your child so they can successfully manage their anxiety. This is a place you can turn for easy-to-understand information, recommendations, support, and a little humor along the way. Because how do you survive parenting without a sense of humor? As we welcome you, we want to take a quick moment to acknowledge that this book is for anyone with a child who experiences anxiety or who works with children who experience anxiety. Actually, we believe this workbook is for everyone because everyone experiences some amount of anxiety sometimes and it's a good thing to know how to manage it! You'll see we use the word "parent" most frequently, but please know that we are not just referring to biological parents; we are including stepparents, adoptive parents, foster parents, LGBTQIA+ family members, grandparents, extended family members, family friends, teachers, babysitters, and anyone else in a child's life who wants to support them.

How to Use This Workbook

This book has five chapters, and we highly recommend that you go through them in order. Although it might be less time consuming to skip straight to the interventions, we recommend that you don't do that. Chapter 1,

"Anxiety: The Basics," is full of important information about what anxiety is and how it may look in your child. We suggest you read that chapter first, as it provides an important framework for everything that comes after.

After the basics comes the hands-on fun stuff: the parent prep and interventions chapters. This is the part of the book where all the action is—literally! In these chapters, we include a number of concrete things that you can *do* to help your family.

It is imperative that you do the important preliminary work in chapter 2, "Parent Prep." There, we challenge you to consider how your thoughts and actions may be contributing to your child's anxiety. Kids do not operate in a vacuum. If you want to see your child gain awareness into their behavior and make some changes, you have to be prepared to do the same. And you may find that engaging in these prep activities will feel good for you!

Chapter 3, "Interventions," provides dozens of activities for your child to try. These activities are designed to help children find some relief from their anxious feelings. If parent prep is the *doing* part for adults, these interventions are the *doing* part for kids. These two chapters include nearly sixty activities to help you accomplish the book's overall goal: helping children manage anxiety. We hope you and your children will find many of them fun and useful.

The final part of the book consists of the maintenance and resources chapters and the appendices. Once you have determined which interventions are helpful for you and your child, you want to maintain the progress you gain! These chapters make that possible.

Limitations

We hate to admit it, but this book has limitations. It is not a replacement for therapy, and it will not diagnose your child. Diagnosis and therapy are best left to professionals. (We'll discuss this more in chapter 1, "The Basics.") This workbook will also not "cure" your child's anxiety. That's not what we're aiming for because, as you'll learn in this book, some anxiety is a good thing.

A Note about COVID-19

When we began work on this book the words "coronavirus," "COVID-19," and "global pandemic" were not a part of our vocabulary. We could never have imagined how different the world would look and feel when we reached the publishing stage. But alas, here we are. You may be wondering if all the information in this book is relevant given our changed reality. We assume this because we wondered the same thing. We gave this concern a lot of thought, and ultimately we feel that no matter what is happening in the world, the relevance of the information in this book hasn't really changed. The topics are just as important, if not more so, now. Perhaps two years ago, you would have sought out this book thinking that only one of your children was anxious or that your child was only dealing with one minor anxiety-related issue. However, now its content may feel applicable for virtually everyone in your family given the changes you all are encountering in your daily lives. This is normal and, quite honestly, to be expected given the global coronavirus crisis. One of the hallmarks of *Working with Worry* is that it's not about pathologizing: we are not trying to diagnose your kid—or you! Instead, our book is about easing anxiety when it is impacting your children and family.

COVID-19 has changed us. As individuals, as a country, and as a world, we are experiencing greater amounts of stress, grief, and loss. All of these factors can interact with anxiety and exacerbate its effects or change how it manifests. That said, it has not necessarily changed the way we intervene to help address anxiety and its effects. Many of the interventions in this book will help you and your loved ones make sense of these complicated emotions. With that in mind, you will not see much direct mention of COVID-19 in this book. This is an intentional decision on our part. While we recognize that this pandemic is a relevant factor, we also believe that the process—doing your own work, helping your child discover coping skills that work for them, and coming up with a maintenance plan—remains the same during the global coronavirus crisis. No matter your personal journey, we believe that the guidance we provide will serve you and your family well.

Thanks for joining us!

Samantha and Melissa

1

Anxiety: The Basics

Chapter Introduction

This chapter is a crash course in what anxiety looks like in children. Most people have a general sense of what anxiety is but aren't sure how it differs from concepts such as worry and shyness. In this chapter, we help you to distinguish between them. We also provide information about the neuroscience of anxiety. Finally, we include general information about child development to give you a sense of what is age appropriate in relation to anxiety, as well as a better sense of when a child's anxiety may be falling outside the bounds of typical.

Though we hope the information provided in this book will help your understanding of anxiety in children, it is *not* a substitute for talking with a mental health professional about your child specifically. We want to help you be able to recognize the signs and symptoms of anxiety, but remember that only a mental health professional can make a diagnosis and/or provide treatment.

Defining Anxiety

People often use the word "anxiety" in a casual or colloquial sense without really understanding its true meaning. Being anxious is related to being worried, stressed, or nervous, but these are not all the exact same concepts. Throughout the book—and especially in the interventions chapter—you will see us refer to worry and stress as opposed to anxiety. This is because worry and stress are common, easily recognizable symptoms of anxiety. Just know that while it is often easiest to identify the worry that one is experiencing, there typically are additional anxiety symptoms happening as well. In an effort to make you aware of these additional symptoms and to clarify how we think about anxiety in a clinical way, we define it for you here.*

What Is Anxiety?

According to the American Psychological Association (APA),[1] anxiety is "an emotion characterized by feelings of tension, worried thoughts, and physical changes such as increased heart rate, rapid breathing, and body tension. People with *anxiety disorders* [emphasis added] usually have recurring thoughts or concerns. They may avoid certain situations out of worry. They may also have physical symptoms such as sweating, trembling, dizziness, or rapid heartbeat."

For example, if your child talks frequently about how scary fire is after witnessing in person a local building burn to the ground, it is likely a reasonable and logical reaction.

---

*This book is a support tool and does not take the place of a professional mental health provider.

It is important to recognize that anxiety can be useful for a child (or anyone). It helps them stay alert in unfamiliar environments. It can sound the alarm when they forget to study for a test. It can prepare the muscles in their body for action in an important game. However, it is not foolproof. The alarm can sound when there is no actual threat as well.

When thinking about anxiety, it's also important to consider context and whether a child's reaction is a reasonable and logical response to what is currently happening or if the response is out of proportion. For example, if your child talks frequently about how scary fire is after witnessing in person a local building burn to the ground, it is likely a reasonable and logical reaction.

Anxiety is different from . . .

❖ **Worry:** Worry is one of the more common symptoms of anxiety, and it involves your thoughts, sometimes referred to as cognition. Sometimes worry can be described as repetitive thoughts or the sense that you cannot get something out of your mind. It can also include a fixation on something bad happening either in general or with regard to a specific situation. Sometimes people use the words "worry" and "anxiety" to mean the same thing, but they are not interchangeable. Unlike worry, anxiety also includes behavioral and/or physical components, which can occur at the same time as worry or instead of worry. Since worry is one of the more common and easily recognizable symptoms of anxiety, we use the term often throughout the book.

❖ **Stress:** Stress is your body's physical response to a specific stressor and is usually short-lived. Anxiety is often a reaction to stress, but anxiety is longer lasting than stress.

❖ **Feeling nervous:** Nervousness is being concerned about a specific situation that has the potential to be scary. Anxiety is broader in scope than nervousness.

❖ **Being shy:** Shyness is being reserved or timid in the company of other people, usually those who are unfamiliar. It is true that being shy may create feelings of worry or tension, but it is normal for kids—and adults—to feel shy sometimes. When that shyness is about everything, all of the time, and reactions are significantly disproportionate to the situation, then anxiety might be at play.

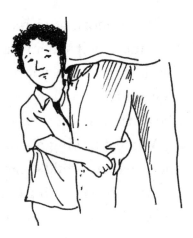

Anxiety is not . . .

❖ **Only for girls:** Although anxiety disorders are diagnosed more frequently in girls and women, they are the most common mental health disorder across genders.[2] Additionally, boys' anxiety is often misdiagnosed or mischaracterized as anger or inattention/hyperactivity.

❖ **Just "growing pains":** All children are shy, stressed, nervous, or worried sometimes. If these feelings are significantly impacting their ability to function or are out of proportion, then they may be anxious, and anxiety is not typically something they will just outgrow.

Anxiety Symptoms

Table 1.1 lists different ways a child or teen may show us that they are anxious. Sometimes symptoms are obvious or verbally stated and sometimes they are communicated through behavior and action (or inaction).

Note that table 1.1 is not meant to serve as a means of diagnosis. Only a mental health professional can diagnose your child with an anxiety disorder.

Table 1.1 Anxiety Symptoms (and How Kids Communicate Them)

Type of Symptom	Examples
Physical	Headaches Stomachaches Vomiting Restlessness Fidgeting Sleep Problems
Anger	Lashing out Yelling Excessive blaming of others "Letting it all out" in a safe space (can be a person or a place) Resisting/rebelling against authority figures (teachers, supervising grown-ups, coaches)
Other Emotional Changes	Extreme sensitivity Frequent/excessive crying Worrying about events far in the future Tantrums or meltdowns that are not age appropriate
Rigidity	Complete inflexibility Demanding that things must be a certain way all the time Overreaction—slight changes lead to meltdowns Strict adherence to very specific routines
Avoidance	Anhendonia (Loss of pleasure in preferred activities/events/people; anhendonia is also a symptom of depression. The reasons why a child is avoiding activities/events/people may clarify whether they are dealing with anxiety or depression.*)

* For example, losing pleasure due to fear (which indicates anxiety) is different than withdrawal due to a lack of interest in pleasurable activities (which indicates depression).

Diagnosing Anxiety

We said it before and we'll say it again: this book is not intended to diagnose your child. Only a mental health professional who has actually met your child can do that. However, we recognize that it may be helpful for parents and teachers to have some sense of diagnostic terms related to anxiety so that if you do consult with a mental health professional, the terms you hear won't be brand new to you. It is also important to note that for any person to meet diagnostic criteria, they must be experiencing a level of distress that is impacting their functioning. In other words, your child may experience anxiety that is not significant enough to require a diagnosis. Remember, we all experience anxiety at times.

Neurobiology: Anxiety and the Brain

Mental health disorders are internal. We can see or feel certain symptoms and related behaviors, but much of what is going on is happening *inside* the body—specifically in the brain and nervous system. Researchers frequently discover more about these interactions, and it is likely our understanding of the relationship between anxiety and the brain will continue to expand. We understand that some people really want to know about the latest research and the science behind what we tell you and others don't. So, in this section we talk just a little about the neuroscience that underlies the material in this book. Folks who want more can find additional information and resources in appendix A, "Understanding Anxiety-Related Structures and Processes."

Anxiety is a response to a *perceived* threat. As such, it begins in the brain and is supported by various parts of the nervous system. You can think of it as the body's built-in alarm system. But there are two catches: (1) we are not always consciously aware of why the alarm is sounding, and (2) sometimes the alarm is going off even when a threat is not real (note our earlier emphasis on *perceived* threat).

Anxiety Quick Facts

Prevalence:

Anxiety disorders are the most common mental health disorder in children and teens.[3]

8% of all children and adolescents experience anxiety disorders.[4]

Approximately 1/3 of adolescents between 13–18 years old experience anxiety disorders.[5]

In teens, the prevalence of anxiety is higher for girls: 38% vs. 26.1% for boys.[6]

The number of anxiety cases diagnosed in childhood increased 17% between 2013–2015.[7]

Median age of onset of anxiety (when it all begins) is 11 years old.[8]

Median age of onset of phobias (fears of specific things) is as young as 7 years old.[9]

The most common anxiety disorders are specific phobia (8.7%) and social anxiety (6.8%).[10]

The most common coexisting disorders (2+ disorders diagnosed at the same time) include depression[11] and ADHD.[12]

Cognitive behavioral therapy (CBT) and medication are both effective treatment options.[13]

Parental involvement improves treatment outcome.[14]

Imagine you are walking in a forest and see a bear. Before you have any real conscious awareness of what's going on, a part of the limbic system in your brain called the amygdala (see p. 161 in appendix A) sends a signal that the animal in front of you is dangerous. It tells you that you'd better do something. This is the fight, flight, or freeze reaction (see p. 163 in appendix A), and it happens fast. The brain observes a potentially dangerous situation, assesses that situation, and reacts accordingly. All of this happens in a matter of milliseconds. It has to. If it takes too long, you may not make it out of the forest!

But now, imagine that you are reacting to a bear . . . even when there is no bear present. That's anxiety. Our brains and nervous systems don't always know the difference between *real* threats and *perceived* threats without some conscious assistance. The human ability to draw the distinction between real and perceived is a survival mechanism. And children cannot always differentiate between the two types of threats—real and perceived—because their brains just aren't mature enough. Distinguishing between the two is hard to do as an adult, so of course a child with a not-fully-developed brain is going to struggle with it! As explained in appendix A, a child's brain continues to develop until they are around twenty-five years old, so your little one's brain is less developed than you may think!

Understanding how the brain and anxiety work allows us to see that a child who feels scared by a person dressed up as a clown, for example, may actually be having the same internal experience they would have face-to-face with a dangerous predator! It also helps us to understand that when we tell kids (or adults for that matter) there's "nothing to be scared of" or "nothing to worry about," it's ineffective and dismissive. For that person, there is very much something to worry about!

For more information and resources on the neuroscience of anxiety, refer to appendix A, "Understanding Anxiety-Related Structures and Processes."

**What Research Tells Us
about Anxiety and the Brain**

An enlarged amygdala (fear center) in
the brain *can increase anxiety.*

A lack of connectivity/integration between
systems within the brain *can increase anxiety.*

An imbalance of neurotransmitters *can increase anxiety.*

The way the amygdala and hippocampus
connect to memories *can increase anxiety.*

Misconceptions about Anxiety

There are many misconceptions about anxiety. Here we debunk some of the more common assumptions. Which one is the most surprising to you?

Misconception: Anxiety is always bad . . .
Fact: *Anxiety is protective.*

Anxiety has helped us survive for centuries by activating our fight, flight, or freeze reaction (see p. 163). Anxiety signals to our brains that we need to do something fast without giving our reaction too much thought. Our goal in this book is to help your child manage anxiety, not eliminate it.

Misconception: *Getting rid of anxiety is the goal . . .*

Fact: *Learning to tolerate anxiety is the goal.*

Anxiety is necessary not only for survival but for ordinary day-to-day life. *We do not want to get rid of anxiety entirely.* Anxiety is what helps motivate us to work on the things that are hard for us. We all knew that one kid in high school who didn't seem to care about anything—never got any work done and hardly ever went to class. A lack of anxiety often means a lack of motivation, which means you never get anything done. So we don't want to eliminate it. Anxiety also has an activating component so it can give your child the energy they need to finish their homework on time, get through a presentation they may feel nervous about, or stay energized for a big game. The goal is to make the anxiety manageable so the child can feel as if they are in control of their anxiety rather than the anxiety being in control of them.

Misconception: *My kid must be the only one going through this . . .*

Fact: *Not so! Your child is not alone!*

Anxiety disorders are the most commonly diagnosed disorders during childhood and adolescence (see Anxiety Quick Facts, p. 11).

Misconception: *I would know if my child were anxious . . .*

Fact: *Kids are shockingly good at hiding their anxiety.*

Anxiety can present in many different ways, especially in children. Additionally, many of the symptoms of anxiety are hidden (such as rapid heartbeat), so you may not be able to see what your child is experiencing. In this book we want to provide you with some tools to be able to recognize the signs and symptoms of anxiety, but remember that only a mental health professional can make a diagnosis and/or provide treatment.

Misconception: *Anxiety and shyness are the same thing . . .*
Fact: *Anxiety is not the same as being shy.*

Anxiety has components to it that occur in a child's mind and body. They can look like shyness on the surface, but they are different. Some people who are shy may also experience anxiety, but shyness and anxiety are not synonymous. Recall from page 7 that *anxiety is different from shyness, nervousness, worry, and stress.*

Child Development: A Quick Primer

In this section, we summarize some of what goes on developmentally as children grow. When we talk about development, we are referring to how children grow and change as they age both physically and psychologically. This is the stuff we don't always think about, but development is ever-present and always happening in our kids. Understanding more about what behaviors are age appropriate is imperative when you are trying to determine how typical your child's anxiety is. For example, a three-year-old feeling afraid of a dark room is very different than a ten-year-old having this same fear. This is not to say a ten-year-old shouldn't be afraid; rather the cause of their fears is likely different because they are at a different developmental stage. At three, a child does a lot of magical thinking and may be scared of monsters in the dark. At ten, children are more aware of their vulnerabilities and real-world dangers, so a fear of the dark may equate to fear of an intruder.

Because of these developmental differences, the fears of each child need to be addressed differently. For example, a parent could help their three-year-old child utilize their magical thinking by helping them imagine one of their stuffed animals vanquishing the evil monster. With a ten-year-old who is scared of someone breaking into the house, you can have a conversation with them about how safe your home and neighborhood are and the steps you have taken to make it even safer (e.g., locks on the door, an alarm system, automatic floodlights). This is only one example, but it illustrates why understanding the developmental context within which your child is operating is so important in understanding and helping with their anxieties.

Should I Be Concerned about My Child's Anxiety?

We've thrown a lot at you so far, and you may be thinking: When is it time to be concerned? How do you know when your child's fears are more than what's considered "normal"? When is it time to seek help?

Generally stated, the following situations may be concerning and could warrant a call to a professional . . .

❖ Your child's fears gain momentum and become worse instead of reducing and becoming less over time.

Maurice is nervous about starting a new school and expresses this concern verbally to his parents about once a day in the weeks leading up to the first day. As school begins and the months go on, Maurice makes many new friends who regularly call and want to hang out with him. However, he continues to express feelings of worry to his parents several times a day.

❖ Your child's worry is always there regardless of who they are with or the setting they are in; the worry never (or rarely) goes away.

> Maya is always concerned about school and her grades. She thinks about it before school, after school, on weekends, and during summer vacation.

❖ The anxiety symptoms are not proportional to the cause; in other words, the concerns are much bigger than they should be based on the problem.

> Ashley is afraid of dogs. She has never had a bad or scary interaction with a dog, but she has always been afraid of them. She will not go to a friend's house if they have pet dogs, she crosses the street when she sees a dog, and she doesn't like seeing pictures or shows about them. Lately, she has even turned down a few trips to the playground and walks in her favorite parks because she's afraid she will see a dog. If her parents try to reassure her she begins to cry, loses her breath, and becomes completely distraught.

❖ The worry is extreme or unrealistic.

> Dylan is afraid of
> storms. Even when it starts
> raining he gets extremely anxious—he
> talks about it nonstop, cries, hides, etc. Even
> on sunny days he is often looking to the sky
> and taking note if clouds are rolling in or if some
> clouds look darker than others. His teachers have
> mentioned that he often gets distracted because
> he seems to be looking out the window during
> lessons. He's a great baseball player but
> has refused to go to some practices
> because of a chance of rain.

❖ Your child's anxiety symptoms significantly impact their everyday functioning or the everyday functioning of significant others (e.g., family members, caregivers).

> Jada does not want to go
> to school in the morning. She refuses to
> eat breakfast, throws things around her room,
> and screams at every member of the household each
> morning. Efforts to calm her down are ignored or lead
> to more screaming. Jada's parents are frequently
> late to work because she misses the
> school bus so often.

Table 1.2 Child Development at a Glance

	Preschool Ages 3–5	School-Aged Ages 5–12	Teenagers Ages 13+
Cognitive Our thoughts	Beginning to distinguish between past and future	Understanding their thoughts are different from others' thoughts	Being self-conscious and moody
Psychosocial Interactions with others	Beginning to assert power and control	Looking for approval from peers and society	Searching for personal identity, values, beliefs
Academic School-related	Early academic learning	Understanding their own weaknesses	Experiencing increased social demands and pressures
Physical Our bodies	Gross and fine motor skill improvement	Continued motor skill development; emergence of clear physical differences among peers	Puberty
Play Enjoyable activities	Magical thinking/ make-believe; exploring their environment	Development of ability to tolerate frustration	Experiencing peer pressure during social activities; Friends/ peers more important than parents
Common Fears Fears that typically occur at this age	The potty The dark Monsters Strangers Shadows Getting lost Bugs/animals Sleeping alone Separation	The dark Monsters/Zombies Toilet issues Scary media Closets Bad weather and weather events Peer rejection Doctor/dentist/ shots Sudden loud noises Bugs/animals	Safety Being home alone Sickness Growing up Peer rejection School/sports/ extracurricular failure School presentation failure Romantic rejection Violence/global current issues (especially older teens)

Table 1.3 lists some examples that illustrate how the symptoms on page 21 may play out in everyday life. Keep in mind that everything is relative and age-dependent. We say it is relative because, for example, if your child exhibits behavior listed in the table as "not a concern" but that behavior is unusual for them, it may still warrant a call to a professional. You know your child best. If you are ever unsure whether something is a concern, call a professional or talk to your child's pediatrician. You can never go wrong with getting a professional opinion.

Getting Help

If, by the time you finish this book, you still have unaddressed concerns and unanswered questions about your child's anxiety, consider calling a professional. We realize, as professionals, that's easy for us to say! But what does that even mean? Where do you start? For more information on whom to call or where to look for help when you do have a concern, please refer to appendix B, "Additional Support and Professional Treatment Options."

Table 1.3: How Concerned Should I Be?

Not a Concern	Keep An Eye on It	Call a Professional
Your 6-year-old mentions something scary that was talked about in school. He talks about it several times over the course of a week, then forgets about it.	Your 6-year-old continues to talk every day about a scary thing he'd heard in school. It is annoying but is not keeping your child from engaging in any normal activities and doesn't seem to be impacting his mood.	Your 6-year-old does not want to go to a certain class or spend time with the teacher because that teacher is the one who introduced a scary topic. Your child's concern about the scary thing has impacted his willingness to participate in certain activities.
Your 8-year-old is worried about a playdate with a new friend. She is especially worried about the playdate right before going. Your child still goes to the playdate and is happy afterward.	Your 8-year-old is worried about a playdate. The night before she has trouble sleeping. She insists on you coming to the playdate and staying at least for a few minutes but then accepts you leaving her and has a great time and requests another one.	Your 8-year-old is so worried about a playdate that she does not sleep for days beforehand. Afterward, she is still distressed and is second-guessing everything she did during the playdate. She refuses another playdate even when she's invited back.
Your 10-year-old shares his concerns and fears with you on occasion when things feel overwhelming.	Your 10-year-old shares a long list of what is bothering him on a daily basis. He reports that everything is equally overwhelming but is still able to get his schoolwork done and enjoy time with his peers.	Your 10-year-old needs your help coping with his stress in every aspect of his life. You are often late for work or need to leave early to help your child manage his emotions.
Your 11-year-old is upset about missing an easy goal in the last soccer game and mentions once or twice that she's worried her teammates will be mad at her.	Your 11-year-old is worried that her teammates, coach, and friends at school will be mad at her for missing a goal and brings it up a few times over the next few days.	Your 11-year-old reports significant stomach pains for two weeks after missing a goal. Her pediatrician reports that nothing is physically wrong.

Continues ›

Table 1.3: How Concerned Should I Be? (*continued*)

Not a Concern	Keep An Eye on It	Call a Professional
Your 15-year-old worries about schoolwork while at school and while doing homework.	Your 15-year-old worries about schoolwork at school, while doing homework, and randomly throughout the day and sometimes wakes up worried about a big assignment.	Your 15-year-old worries about schoolwork constantly. Even when doing fun activities, he can't seem to stop thinking about the work that needs to be done later.

This Is So Important!

We talk about anxiety in a general way because everyone experiences anxiety. However, when a child's anxiety is so severe that it impacts their ability to function, they may be diagnosed with an anxiety-related mental health disorder. Keep in mind that the information included here is only to inform and help you better understand anxiety. Do not diagnose your child or "guess" at what they may be experiencing. If you feel your child may be struggling significantly, ***seek out a mental health professional.***

Parent Prep: Help Yourself to Help Your Child

Chapter Introduction

Welcome to parent prep! This is the *most important chapter* in our workbook. We are guessing you purchased this book thinking exclusively about your child's anxieties and not giving a second thought to your own. (Isn't that parenthood?) Well, we're here to tell you that we cannot entirely separate those two things: your child's anxieties and your own feelings. For this reason, we have an entire chapter dedicated to focusing on your own relationship with anxiety.

That said, before you start blaming yourself for your child's struggles, we want to remind you that we as parents do not have total control over who our children become. Wow, even just that thought can be anxiety provoking! But it's true. Children are influenced and impacted by friends, television, movies, video games, teachers, social media, and their environment. Many children experience traumatic life events or losses that are well beyond parental control. Then, of course, there is also genetic makeup and predisposition to consider. So, while parents do play a critical role, we don't want to imply that you have total control over your child's experience of anxiety. We do, however, believe you have a great deal of power in supporting your children and helping them navigate their anxiety.

And you are ahead of the game. You are reading this book, and that means you already recognize that your child needs some support and you are taking the steps to provide that support. For that, give yourself a giant pat on the back. Now take a deep breath and dig into your own stuff. This self-exploration will be helpful in understanding, relating to, and ultimately supporting your child.

Parent Self-Reflection

It's important to do your own work on anxiety prior to implementing interventions for your child. To that end, we ask you to consider the following questions:

❖ What is it like for others to be around you when you're anxious? Parents model behavior for children all the time. What are your children learning when they are watching you deal with your own emotions and anxiety?

❖ At the times when your child's anxiety is heightened, what experience of anxiety are *you* having?

❖ Research tells us that anxiety can have a genetic component. Is this the case in your family?

All these questions point to something you may have been thinking in the back of your head but were too afraid to say out loud. And that thought may look something like this: "I need to do something about *my* anxiety before I can help my kid."

The more aware you are of your own anxieties, how they manifest, and how to manage them, the more easily you will be able to support your child in managing their anxieties. In this chapter, we help you examine your own anxiety. The purpose of this examination is not to point blame but to raise awareness. You will learn what some of *your* anxieties are about, how they may be impacting you, and how they may be affecting your child. We give you tools, language, and resources to help you manage your own anxiety. (In fact, to be honest, all the activities in this book, even the ones that are tailored to children, are tools you can use too!) Also in this chapter, we ask you to think about whether it may be helpful to talk to others about your child's anxiety as you consider all the ways to provide support. Finally, we introduce the idea of KYST parent behaviors and language. Curious what KYST is? Read on!

To get started, you need to consider your own anxiety. Completing Activity 2.1 is a first step toward better understanding how you are feeling, what you are doing with those feelings, and how that may be influencing your child's anxiety.

Activity 2.1: Parent Activity

Anxiety Self-Reflection

Part 1

Write the answers to the questions in the blanks below. Feel free to complete your answers on another sheet of paper if you need more room.

1. How do I experience my anxiety—physically and emotionally? *How does your body feel and what is going on inside your head when you are feeling anxious?*

   _____

   _____

   _____

   _____

2. How may my manifestations of anxiety be perceived by my child? *This question is related to the question above. What do your children see or feel when you are experiencing anxiety? Can they see or hear or feel what is happening when your anxiety occurs?*

_____

_____

_____

_____

3. Do I have a family history of anxiety? *You may be aware of a family member who has a diagnosis of anxiety or you may have heard from family members or observed behavior that a family member struggles with anxiety. We don't want you to diagnose your family members here! Just consider whether there may be a genetic component that you had not considered before.*

_____

_____

_____

_____

4. How do my family of origin and my extended family handle anxiety? *All families experience stressors. When your family of origin went through a stressful time and family anxiety may have been elevated, can you recall how it was handled?*

_____

_____

_____

_____

Part 2

5. Identify the stressors you consider to be the most challenging for you right now and use those to answer the questions that follow. We've listed some common topics for you to circle here, but feel free to add your own.

Work Concerns	Health Issues	Trauma	Parenting
Marriage and Family Concerns	Grief and Loss	Financial Stressors	

Other Concerns:

_____

_____

_____

Answer the following questions for each concern you circled or wrote in above:

6. What is the current narrative I am telling myself about this concern? *The narrative is the story you tell yourself about this concern. Think about how you talk to yourself and others about it. For example, if a project at work did not go as well as anticipated, do you tell yourself that you are a failure, are going to lose your job, and will likely never find another? Or are you able to see multiple reasons for why this particular thing didn't go as planned and direct your focus toward the next project?*

_____

_____

_____

_____

7. What are the feelings I have related to this
    concern? *Concerning the examples you iden-
    tified in the previous questions, are your feel-
    ings directed inward? Are you having negative
    feelings toward yourself? Or do you have
    negative feelings about the task itself? Which
    of these feelings do you feel more strongly?*

Calm, Angry, Scared, Irritated, Annoyed, Confused, Sad, Surprised, Happy, Relieved, Cautious, Bored, Exhausted, Ashamed, Surprised, Embarrassed, Curious, Lonely, Overwhelmed

_____

_____

_____

_____

8. What mood(s) am I experiencing while dealing with this concern?

_____

_____

_____

_____

9. What behaviors (actions or inactions, interactions with others) do I
   engage in as a result of this concern? *For example, in the work example,
   do you stay at work much later than you would otherwise to show
   how hard you are working? Are you checking in more often with your
   manager to get reassurance? Are you retreating and avoiding projects
   you otherwise would have wanted to work on?*

_____

_____

_____

_____

10. What types of things do I say around, or directly to, my child as a reaction to this concern? *Are you less playful than you were prior to this situation? Are you more likely to talk about financial concerns or set limits with your children around things that you were otherwise carefree about?*

_____

_____

_____

_____

Again, be sure to answer the questions in part 2 for all concerns that you circled above.

Part 3

Consider three common things that we *all* do as parents: project, helicopter, and criticize. Anxiety projections are a defense mechanism in which a person puts anxious feelings onto someone else unintentionally. For example, if you are anxious about large gatherings, you assume your child will be nervous about going to birthday parties and project this feeling onto them. Helicopter parenting is when a parent is overly protective or takes an excessive interest in the life of a child. The idea is that a parent is hovering so much around their child (like a helicopter) that it is difficult for the child to solve their own problems or make their own decisions. Critical language refers to speaking to your child in a way that indicates their faults or expresses disapproval and judgment.

We're not being accusatory. We assume you do these things from time to time because we're all human. We do them too—every parent does! It may be hard to admit that we all do these things, but it is so important to be honest with yourself here. With honesty comes awareness, and awareness is the first step toward making the changes you want and need to make. You can do it!

Write the answers to the questions in the blanks below. Feel free to complete your answers on another sheet of paper if you need more room.

Anxiety Projection

11. In general, what causes anxiety for me? (Review your answers in part 2 of the activity.)

_____

_____

_____

_____

12. Are there ways I might be trying to protect my child from things that cause anxiety for me?

_____

_____

_____

_____

13. How may my efforts at protection be affecting my child?

_____

_____

_____

_____

Helicopter Parenting

14. Am I a helicopter parent? In what ways?

_____

_____

_____

_____

15. How may I be negatively affecting my child by trying to protect him/her?

_____

_____

_____

_____

Excessive Criticism

16. How often do I correct or redirect my child's behavior? *Your initial response may be "hardly ever," but we urge you to really think about this one. Check in with yourself the next few days as you help with homework, ask for assistance with chores, reprimand problematic behavior, etc.*

_____

_____

_____

_____

17. Do I ever speak to my child in ways that I don't feel good about?

_____

_____

_____

_____

18. How may my criticism be affecting my child?

_____

_____

_____

_____

Part 4

As you answered the questions in this worksheet, you may have thought of something we didn't address.

19. What else may be going on in my life that could have an impact on the way my child interprets or experiences stress in our home?

_____

_____

_____

_____

20. How may this be affecting my child?

_____

_____

_____

_____

You are off to a great start just by thinking through the previous questions and being honest with yourself. As you continue to work through this workbook, try to keep your answers in this activity at the forefront of your mind and consider the implications for yourself and your child.

Of course, just thinking through the items on the anxiety reflection can be anxiety provoking. You may be thinking, "Oh my gosh! I must be ruining my child and causing all of their anxiety!" But hold on there. It is true that as a parent, you—and your emotions—affect your child's manifestation of anxious feelings. But this also means that you can influence things the other way! You have the power to help your child cope. To do that you need to find interventions that work for you so you can manage your own anxiety more effectively. The next chapter is full of these. And you also can learn to model more regulated language and behaviors so you can start to separate your child's anxiety from your own. We call these behaviors KYST, and we will introduce them next.

KYST Parent Behaviors and Language

Now that you have thought about your own anxieties, it may be more clear where your anxiety and your child's anxiety intersect. This section will help you figure out what to do with your newly discovered awareness. Making some simple changes in your language and behavior to engage in what we call KYST behaviors is a great first step. What does KYST stand for? Keep Your Stuff Together.

As parents, we have all had "those" days when keeping it together can be really hard work—borderline impossible. This section is intended to help you learn to release some of your own anxiety. The hope is that if you, as the parent, can reduce your anxiety, that may in turn reduce the anxieties everyone in the family is experiencing. The exercises on the next few pages address some of the most common ways we tend to perpetuate anxiety and challenge you to do a few things differently.

One of those things we encourage you to do is develop greater self-awareness. But once you are self-aware, what do you do about it? At the end of the chapter we talk about ways for you to find your own support (see p. 56). Perhaps this involves engaging more intentionally in self-care activities. Perhaps it means spending more time with friends or calling family members more often. It can also mean seeking professional support in the form of your own therapy. Once you go through all the activities, we hope that you start thinking about which forms of support will be most helpful to you. We encourage you to have an open mind because, in some ways, getting your own support—formal or informal—is the hardest part! In the end, you are worth it—trust us.

KYST parenting is the idea that you are operating from a self-regulated state. It means that you are in control of what you are thinking and saying and not simply being reactive, punitive, or dismissive—reactions that are especially easy to have when tired, overwhelmed, or overworked.

How many times have you said no, yelled, or given a consequence and then realized later that your reaction wasn't well thought out? For example, maybe in a moment of anger you took away screen time for the next year! Maybe you would have made a different choice if you had just taken a deep breath or counted to ten before responding to your child.

Now, to be clear, all parents do this every once in a while, but as loving parents, we want to keep it to a minimum. We want to feel that our choices are reasonable and rational. We want to look back at our choices and feel that we made the best possible decision at the time. A decision that we don't later regret. That's KYST. It's recognizing how our own thoughts, feelings, and behaviors influence our parenting choices.

KYST involves the following:

❖ Honest self-reflection

❖ Willingness to let your child fail

❖ Acceptance: your child is not you and you are not your child

❖ Talking things out

❖ Modeling problem solving

❖ Choosing your words carefully

In this chapter we will discuss each of these steps and help you put KYST into action.

Honest Self-Reflection

Sometimes as parents it feels instinctive to meet our child's needs before our own. But that strategy is actually not as helpful as it seems. Taking care of your own issues first is the equivalent of putting on your oxygen mask on the plane before helping your child with theirs. Until you are able to breathe, you're not really in a position to help someone else do it. The exercises and interventions in Activity 2.2 are a great place to start if you are looking for ideas on how you can nurture yourself, reduce stress, and learn to manage your anxiety—no matter what's going on. When you do these things, you are practicing KYST.

Activity 2.2: Parent Activity

Anxiety Mind and Body Cues

Answer the following prompts about how your stress manifests and what you do to reduce your anxiety. For each one, circle all those that apply.

1. When I feel anxious, I notice these changes in my body:

Sweaty palms	Racing heart	Muscle tension	Jaw tightening
Increased irritability	Pressure in my chest	Feeling on edge	Headaches
Upset stomach	Butterflies	Feeling jittery	

Other:

---

2. When I feel anxious, I notice these changes in my thoughts:

   Obsessing   Negative outlook   Lower mood

3. Tools I use to fight off these physical manifestations of anxiety include:

   Exercise   Downtime   Progressive muscle   Deep breathing
                                       relaxation

4. Tools I use to fight off these cognitive manifestations of anxiety (i.e.,
   anxious thoughts) include:

   Positive   Talking to   Time with   Time with
   self-talk   others   friends   family

   Meditations   Exercise   Therapy   Taking walks

Willingness to Let Your Child Fail

We're going to give you some advice: *allow your child to fail.* Although reading this statement may almost physically hurt you as a parent, the truth is, life is full of failures, rejections, and losses, and kids need to learn how to deal with them. Let your child fail and experience frustration when it is safe to do so (this means letting them try out for a sports team with no guarantee of making the roster, *not* dive headfirst into the deep end of an unfamiliar swimming pool).

Exposure to failure will help your child realize that when they do fail, it's not the end of the world. It will help to remind you of that very important fact too. And of course, you will be there to support them in their sadness and encourage them when they're ready to try again. Remember that KYST parenting means that you are working on supporting your child's experience of the situation, not experiencing it as your own! As you complete Activity 2.3, you can choose a scenario that has already occurred or one that you fear happening in the future.

Activity 2.3: Parent Activity

Fear of (Your Child's) Failure

1. Circle the events listed below that your child has experienced.

   My child made mistakes in front of others while participating in an activity.

   My child was not selected for something they were hoping to be chosen for (a play, a team, an academic opportunity).

   My child has physical or emotional limitations that make some of the hopes we had for them unrealistic.

   Other: _____

   _____

Answer the following questions:

2. What aspects of my child's failure was uncomfortable for me?

   _____

   _____

   _____

   _____

3. Did any aspect of my child's failure bother me more than it bothered my child?

   _____

   _____

   _____

   _____

4. What was the eventual outcome of my child's experience of failure?

_____

_____

_____

_____

5. Was my child's experience of failure helped or hurt by my reaction to the failure?

_____

_____

_____

_____

6. Were there any ways that I struggled to keep my stuff together (KYST)? Did I do or say anything that I would prefer to change next time?

_____

_____

_____

_____

Acceptance: Your Child Is Not You and You Are Not Your Child

Sometimes as parents we project our own feelings on our children. It is not a problem to encourage your child to try something that you find/found enjoyable, but it is important to be careful that you are not insisting on them participating in something just because it was your thing. (For a classic example of this, watch the movie *Varsity Blues*.) Likewise, just because you may have had a bad experience doing something, you don't want to suppress your kids' interests in that same thing. Think about the activities you loved, what you hated, and what your parents pushed you to do or wouldn't allow you to do and consider how your own passions and failures may be related to your reaction and decisions around your child's activities.

Activity 2.4: Parent Activity

Shifting Assumptions

1. What were my favorite activities as a child? Be as specific as possible.

   _____

   _____

   _____

   _____

2. What types of things was I afraid of as a child?

   _____

   _____

   _____

   _____

3. What activities did I not do as a child (for any reason: fear, finances, access, etc.) but wish that I had?

   _____

   _____

   _____

   _____

4. What activities did I do as a child solely because my parents wanted me to?

_____

_____

_____

_____

5. What activities would I like my child to participate in (or steer clear of)? How are these activities related to the activities I listed in response to the previous questions?

_____

_____

_____

_____

6. What would it mean—for me and/or my child—if my child did not participate in the activities that I want them to (or vice versa)?

_____

_____

_____

_____

7. On a scale from 1 (easy) to 5 (difficult), how able am I to disconnect my feelings about these activities with my child's level of interest?

_____

_____

_____

_____

Talking Things Out

Talking out loud about problems or concerns you are having in your life can be a great tool, and you can model this tool for your children. Of course, we don't want to put our worries on our kids, but letting them know that grown-ups also have struggles we need to work through can be important for kids to see. If they witness you regularly talking about how to manage your own issues, your child will learn how they can problem-solve in their own life. Use the framework listed here and get talking! These steps are not rigid, so don't stress if you miss one; they are thought starters meant to help you navigate the various important pieces of the process.

Steps to Take When You Talk Out a Problem

1. *Pick the problem.* Choose a problem that is relatively benign. Don't share anything that is overwhelming, scary, or otherwise inappropriate for a child. Your problem should be something they can relate to in their own life. Some good kid-appropriate examples are frustration with a coworker speaking over you at a meeting, wondering if a close friend is mad at you, feeling overwhelmed with the amount of work you have to do, or confusion about a task you were given at work. Some not-so-kid-appropriate examples are worries about witnessing your boss harassing someone, concern about a friend who is being abused by a significant other, or doubts about the capability of your child's coach.

2. *State the problem clearly.* State what the issue is in terms your child will understand. Talk about what you feel and what you know. Be as factual as possible.

3. *Express your feelings or opinion.* Name how you feel about what is going on and how it is impacting you.

4. ***Talk about the problem from another perspective.*** State how other people may see the issue.

5. ***List potential solutions.*** List a few things you could do to help resolve the issue. Remember, you are modeling for your child, so even if it feels like there are no solutions, try to come up with something. Who knows? You may surprise yourself!

6. ***Choose one solution to try (and one backup solution).*** Talk about what you are going to do for your next step and why you think that is the route to the best solution. If applicable, choose a backup solution. This reinforces the idea of alternatives and choices for your child.

7. ***Follow up.*** You don't have to act on the solution in front of your child. This is not always possible or appropriate. But if you do act on it, try to remember to tell your child how it went. After all of this listening, they are likely curious! It also closes the loop on the problem-solving process.

Review this example script and then try using these steps to talk about a real problem in your life in Activity 2.5.

Example Script for Talking Out a Problem:

The problem: You are worried that a friend at work is angry with you.

Sample script: I've noticed lately that Taylor and I haven't been talking at work as much. We used to talk every morning, but now, when I arrive she is at her desk staring at her computer screen [state the problem]. I'm feeling like she doesn't want to hang out and she may be angry at me because I was late for her big presentation last week [your feelings]. Things have been busy at work so she may just be really busy, or maybe she feels like she's more productive when she first gets to work so she wants to cut down on distractions in the morning [different perspectives]. I wonder what I should do. Maybe I can write her an email and invite her to lunch. I could also just stop by her office tomorrow morning to say hi and check in quickly. Or I could just leave it alone and wait for her to talk to me [three possible solutions]. I think I'll write an email and invite her to lunch. If anything needs to be said, we can do it at lunch away from the office [pick a solution]. If that doesn't work, I'll just drop by her office [pick a backup solution]. I'll write that email as soon as I get to the office tomorrow.

Sample follow-up: (A few days later) So I emailed Taylor and we went to lunch today. She was a little hurt about my being late to her presentation, and I explained that I had an emergency that morning that made me late. She had noticed I wasn't there, but that wasn't the whole reason we haven't been talking as much. She has also been really busy with work and has been putting her energy into a new project.

Activity 2.5: Parent Activity
Talking Out a Problem

The problem:_____

_____

_____

Script (bullet points are fine): _____

_____

_____

_____

_____

Follow-up:_____

_____

_____

Modeling Problem Solving

In Activity 2.5, we discussed talking problems out, but what is also being modeled is problem solving. Now that you've challenged yourself to talk through a problem constructively, try talking through a problem your child is having and helping them to navigate through the same steps you just did. Remember, you are not doing it *for* them. You are asking questions and helping them do it themselves, the same way the book just did with you.

Activity 2.6: Parent Activity

Promoting Problem Solving

1. Ask your child to pick a problem and state it to you.

2. Ask your child if their problem is small, medium, or big.

3. Ask your child to express their feelings about the problem. Remind them of some common feelings if they are having trouble defining or expressing their feelings.

4. Restate their problem back to them and validate their feelings about it.

5. Ask them if they've considered another point of view. If they haven't, ask them to think of one now. Offer suggestions of possible alternative views if they have trouble thinking of them.

6. Ask them to consider possible solutions for their problem.

7. Restate their possible solutions and let them know you trust them to choose the best one.

8. Suggest they implement one of their choices and then follow up with you to tell you what happened.

Activity 2.6 may seem like it belongs in the next chapter, where the interventions for your kids are, but this exercise is actually about how parents can learn how to let kids handle things themselves, even when it's difficult for us to do that. And remember, if things don't go as planned and your child's first solution does not solve the problem, you still need to praise your child for trying and encourage them to think through different approaches they can try next time. This can increase your child's belief in their ability to handle difficult situations.

Choosing Your Words Carefully

Words are powerful. Sometimes the things we say to our children stick! In Activity 2.7, we consider various ways that our words can have a big impact on our kids. Here we encourage you to reflect on the words you are already using and where you can start to introduce more positive communication. Keep in mind that it is not always the words themselves but the *way* you use them that has the biggest impact. Check out the following tips for guidance:

Activity 2.7: Parent Activity
Words Are Powerful

KYST Parent Language

1. *Validate!* Who doesn't love to feel understood? Feeling heard, validated, and accepted makes it easier for children (and adults) to move through whatever they are facing. Words like "I hear you," "I get it," and "that makes sense" can be so empowering for kids to hear from their parents—or anyone! Take a few minutes to list the things you can say to let your child know that what they are experiencing is real and that you understand.

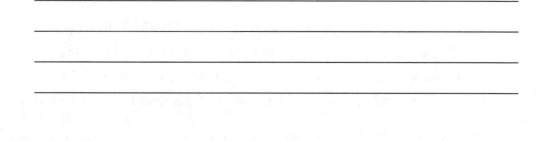

_____

_____

_____

_____

2. *Share your perspective.* Once someone feels heard and validated, that experience often allows them to be open to other ideas and perspectives. Let your child in on *your* experience of the situation. Use language that shows curiosity and supports problem solving and information gathering. This encourages your child to think about it and come to their own conclusion, therefore increasing feelings of competence and confidence.

Consider the following sentence starters and complete the thought in relation to something that your child recently experienced. Think about a recent conversation with your child. How could you have shared your thoughts without telling them how to act or feel?

Examples of Positive Ways to Share your Perspective
Complete these sentences in your own words.

"Here's how I see it: _____

_____

_____ "

"Another way to think of that might be: _____

_____

_____ "

"I'm wondering if _____

_____

is also true. What do you think?"

3. *Eliminate "but," "however," and "should."* Using "but" or "however" after validating a child often completely negates what you were trying to say, and any feelings of pride or accomplishment are diminished. Using "should" frequently makes children (and adults) feel disempowered,

as they are taken out of the problem-solving equation and just told what to do. For example, if you say, "I love that you remembered to grab your backpack without a reminder this morning, but you forgot your coat again," or, "It's great that you got an A on your project, but you should also be getting As on your tests," you are expressing disappointment and creating shame. Truly, these words are the worst, but they are so easy to fall back on (like we did just then). No matter your intention, these words should be avoided at all costs. (We did it again—argh!) We suggest treating the validation and the perspective sharing as two different sentences. How can you move from validation to perspective sharing? It can feel awkward, so try to practice it with the sample starters we provide here. It's harder than it may sound, so practice as much as you can until it begins to feel like second nature to use words other than "but," "however," and "should."

Think about a recent conversation with your child. How can you talk constructively and avoid negating their voice or telling them how to act?

Example: "I hear you. [pause] Have you thought about it from this perspective?"

Complete these phrases in your own words.

"I get it, _____

_____."

"That's upsetting, _____

_____."

"I had a different thought when you told me about _____

_____."

"_____

and I wonder if there is any other explanation for what happened?"

4. *Use a positive tone of voice.* The tone you use is a big factor in how your child (or anyone else) interprets your words. You can validate and offer perspective, but if your child can sense worry, sarcasm, or annoyance in your voice, your good efforts will all go out the window. With younger children, it may be appropriate to speak in a singsong voice—the kind of upbeat, chipper, sweet voice you use with babies. This soothing singsong tone may not be good to use with tweens and teens. Instead, use an age-appropriate approach that feels natural and upbeat. Make sure your tone is genuine and natural, not forced, because your kids will know if it is. Practice the positive voice with a friend, partner, or family member. You can even practice this voice at work. When you are talking about anything that may be difficult for you, practice the voice and it will soon become second nature when you use it with your kids.

5. *Be honest.* Honesty is really important—especially for tweens and teens who can smell insincerity from a mile away. Be honest about your challenges and your experiences. If you feel a little nervous about an event in your child's life or have gone through something similar, let your child know that. And don't stop there. Let them also know how you overcame your anxiety, or tell them about something you wish you had done differently when you experienced something similar. Getting an honest story from you and learning that you have been through something similar may help your child stop catastrophizing and start problem solving. Below, list some experiences or emotions you have intentionally held back from your kids that you now think could be helpful to share.

Example: When I took my driving test for my license, I was really nervous. I felt overwhelmed and was telling myself negative thoughts. I hit the curb when I was parallel parking and failed the test. The second time I took the test, I had practiced parallel parking a lot and felt ready. I told myself that I would pass—and I did!

_____

_____

_____

_____

Committing to Change

At this point, we hope you have a better sense of how you may be influencing your child's anxiety and ways that you can shift your influence to a more positive one. Hopefully you are realizing that KYST behaviors are an important piece in supporting your child and modeling how they can keep their own stuff together. Activity 2.8 asks you to commit to doing small things differently in order to help yourself and your child. One of the best ways to stick to a change is to write down the change you want to make. Studies have shown that this helps you really commit to it.[1]

Activity 2.8: Parent Activity

Doing Things Differently: Practicing KYST Parenting

Write down a few things you would like to do differently and prioritize them. *Do not attempt to do all of them at once!* Start with one change and work on that one only. Once you feel you have mastered it, move on to the next one. Keep going until you've made the changes you want to. You may just surprise yourself with how easy it becomes.

Examples:

Instead of *telling my seven-year-old the answer to her math homework when she tells me it is hard*, I will try *willingness to let my child fail to encourage her to work through it on her own.*

Instead of *telling my seven-year-old the answer to his math homework when he tells me it is hard*, I will try *modeling problem solving in the hopes of motivating him to ask his teacher for help tomorrow.*

Now try a few on your own. For each of the things you plan to try, pick one of the strategies below and explain how you will implement it to help your child work through an anxiety-provoking event. For a quick refresher, the strategies are:

❖ Honest self-reflection

❖ Willingness to let your child fail

❖ Acceptance: your child is not you and you are not your child

❖ Talking things out

❖ Modeling problem solving

❖ Choosing your words carefully

Instead of _____

_____,

I will try_____

_____.

Instead of _____

_____,

I will try_____

_____.

Instead of _____

_____,

I will try_____

_____.

The previous part of this exercise has you thinking about how to practice KYST parenting. Now that you have a sense of what it looks and sounds like, we want you to challenge yourself by making the commitment to use it! Fill in the blanks below and sign the pledge. Once you sign something, it feels more real. You're officially moving into KYST parenting!

I, [enter your name here] _____, commit to trying these new behaviors or language patterns to help myself and my child. I will keep trying even when it is hard. I will seek support from the following individuals: _____, _____, and _____ as needed. I will not attempt to focus on more than one new behavior or language pattern at a time so I do not overwhelm myself. I am committed and I believe I will succeed!

_____   _____

Your Signature   Witness

Involving Others

If your child is experiencing anxiety that you can see at home, that anxiety is likely affecting them in other areas of their life. By going through this workbook, you are doing your part to provide support at home. But what about when your child is at school, practice, rehearsal, or day care? Who are the other significant adults in your child's life, and what do they need to know? On one hand, it may be best for other adults working with your child to be aware of their need for extra support. On the other hand, you want to be thoughtful about how much you share. Remember that this is your child's personal business and though it includes you, it is not yours. You don't want to share information about your child that would upset or embarrass them. And once you share information about your child, you can't take it back. Activity 2.9 is designed to help you determine why and when to reach out, to whom, and what exactly you want to say.

You don't need to share every detail with other people in your child's life. You may just want to provide a general sense of what is going on, and perhaps the more prominent symptom(s) you have seen, so they know what to be aware of.

Before you decide to talk to someone, think about why you want to talk to this person. Are the anxiety symptoms you see at home ones that manifest physically (for example, your child scratches her hands when nervous and sometimes breaks the skin) and you are worried that an adult needs to know about these symptoms to keep your child safe? Have you noticed that your child's anxiety symptoms seem heightened when they are with this person? (For example, your high schooler has trouble eating dinner each time they have drama practice with a particular teacher.) Or is this person someone you hope will be able to tell you whether they see similar anxiety-related behaviors when they are with your child?

If so, you may want to reach out to this person for help. Perhaps you think this person has found a helpful strategy that you can also use. Or if you are doing some things at home you think would be helpful in this other area, you may want to share them. For example, if you provide a signal to your child to take deep breaths at home, their teacher or coach may want to do the same. That said, first consider if the methods you are suggesting are doable in other settings.

And think about how much you want your child to know about your conversations about them with others. Letting children know you're discussing them with other adults can be helpful in some situations. If you do decide to share that you are talking about them, make sure your child knows that this all about supporting them and making them feel comfortable. Of course, there may also be circumstances where you think conversations are best kept between you and the other adult.

Activity 2.9: Parent Activity

Consulting with Others

1. Whom do I feel I should talk to?

   _____

   _____

   _____

   _____

2. Why does it feel important to me to talk to this person?

   _____

   _____

   _____

   _____

3. What do I want the outcome of sharing information about my child with this person to be and why?

   _____

   _____

   _____

   _____

4. What specific concern(s) do I feel I need to convey? *You don't need to share every detail; you may just want to provide a general sense of what*

is going on, and perhaps the more prominent symptom(s) that you have seen, so they know what to look for.

_____

_____

_____

_____

5. Are there any downsides or risks of sharing this information about my child? *For example, will this embarrass your child? Will your child no longer trust this adult you shared the information with? Are you concerned that the adult (such as a teacher) will treat your child differently or share the information with others?*

_____

_____

_____

_____

6. Do I want to ask for input or suggestions from the person with whom I am sharing the information? *Is this someone who may be able to provide you with additional information about how to approach the anxiety symptoms you see or a different perspective about what might be driving your child's behavior? Perhaps this person has found a helpful intervention that you can also use.*

_____

_____

_____

_____

7. Do I want to share what we are doing at home to address my child's anxiety? *If you are doing some activities that help your child cope with their anxiety symptoms at home that you think would be helpful in this other area, you may want to share them, such as providing your child with a squeeze toy (p. 111) or allowing them to have worry time (p. 65). These examples and many others are explained in detail in the next chapter. That said, first consider if the interventions you are suggesting are doable in other settings.*

8. Do I want to talk to my child about the fact that I will have a conversation about their anxiety issues with this person? If so, what do I want to tell my child?

    _____

    _____

    _____

    _____

9. Do I want there to be a plan for follow-up?

    _____

    _____

    _____

    _____

Finding Support for *Your* Anxiety

Congratulations! If you worked your way through this entire chapter, you are a superstar! We hope you were able to reflect and learn more about your own anxiety through completing these activity worksheets. If, in doing so, you have come to realize that maybe your anxiety is having more of an impact on your family than you originally thought, good for you for seeing your role in the family dynamics.

Recall the exercise about taking care of yourself first in Activity 2.2, Anxiety Mind and Body Cues. We have some suggestions to help you do just that. As we've mentioned, the interventions in the next chapter are not just for kids. As you read through them to determine what may help your child, also try to find the ones that work for you. And if you want to seek out additional information for yourself or if you think you may be interested in seeking therapy, please see appendix B, "Additional Support and Professional Treatment Options."

3

Interventions: Strategies and Coping Activities for Your Child

Chapter Introduction

This chapter provides the actual steps you can take to help and support your child at home. It includes fifty interventions, strategies, and coping skills for your child to try. All the activities are created to help your child better understand their anxiety and to feel empowered to be able to work through it. Fifty is a lot, and you don't have to try all of them. Instead, we recommend starting by picking a few that seem like they may be a good fit for your child and trying those out. We've listed a few of our top picks in table 3.1 if you're looking for some recommendations. If they work, great. If not, try a few others. This process is not one size fits all.

You don't have to approach this rigidly. It isn't necessary that you sit down with an agenda of getting through four exercises in a set amount of time. You can be creative with how you present these activities to your child. For example, you might suggest trying something new as a family over dinner or presenting a few interventions as a game rather than a chore. If all else fails, try one or two when you're in the car!

This chapter begins with a quick anxiety self-reflection for your child to complete (see Activity 3.1). Then we move into four categories of interventions: cognitive restructuring, mindfulness, self-regulation, and creativity.

❖ *Cognitive restructuring* is challenging oneself to think about something in a different way.

❖ *Mindfulness* is bringing a different level of awareness to what's happening in your body or mind and being fully present in the moment.

❖ *Self-regulation* is managing feelings and impulses that may be disruptive to you or other people.

❖ *Creativity* is using art or other outlets to reduce stress.

Note that we group interventions into these broad categories as a way to organize the chapter, but there is some overlap among categories. For example, mindfulness exercises also help with self-regulation, and some of the exercises in creativity may also fit into the mindfulness category.

This chapter also provides age-appropriate guidelines for each intervention. Most of the instructions are written so that a child can read them and follow along. However, some activities have instructions for parents instead, as they are more suitable for little ones who may not be reading yet. Additionally, although many kids will be able to read the instructions, they still might need help fully understanding the concept or premise. Much of this content will be brand new information for kids!

Also, keep in mind that these age guidelines are not meant to be prescriptive—we are not telling you exactly which interventions work with children of certain ages. Instead, we intend these to serve as loose guidelines about when an intervention might be right for your child. Even if something seems babyish and is appropriate for toddlers, your tween may love it and find it really helpful. Also, keep in mind that many of these interventions can be tailored to meet the specific age or interest of your

Table 3.1 Some Favorite Interventions

Samantha's Top Picks!		Melissa's Top Picks!
Daily Mood Record, p. 68		Reframing, p. 84
Sensory Awareness, p. 102		The "So What?" Game, p. 93
Cold Drink of Water, p. 114		Sensory Awareness, p. 102
Anxiety in Your Body, p. 122		Just Listen (or Sing Too), p. 117
Exploring Your Anxiety, p. 124		Count Five Sounds, p. 103

child. *All* of the interventions can work for many different children, but it is important to select ones that are right for your child (or better yet, have them choose).

Remember, the goal here is to have your child start to better understand their anxiety and to feel empowered to be able to work through it. The interventions in this chapter are designed to help with this process.

Tips for Getting the Most Out of the Interventions

There is a lot of information in this chapter, and we do not want you to feel overwhelmed. Table 3.2 suggests a few dos and don'ts when considering which interventions might work best for your child.

Though we felt it would be helpful to include these dos and don'ts, we also want to acknowledge that there really are no hard-and-fast rules as you explore and work through this chapter. Each child is different, and what they need is different. As you try out these interventions, feel free to alter them so they are more to your or your child's liking. Keep going until you find something that you and your child enjoy—and something that works!

Many of these interventions are best if used at home. Others are easy to use at school or other places. We recommend finding at least two go-to techniques from the list of interventions. Ideally, at least one of them will be something that can be done anywhere. As you will see, some of the interventions require supplies or a specific setting. When anxiety is heightened,

Table 3.2 Getting the Most Out of the Interventions

Do	Don't
Identify several possible interventions that could work for your child There are many options, and the interventions are grouped by age and area of interest. Pick a few (one to three) from various sections to try. You never know what your child might like.	**Try all the interventions right away** Start with one at a time (two or three at the most). There is no rush! It is better to find something your child enjoys and will stick with than to try several at once, become overwhelmed, and quit before any of the interventions have a chance to really work.
Suggest different options to your child or allow them to choose Encourage your child to feel some ownership over this process. Talk about why you are doing this, and offer some suggestions for interventions that you think might help. Let them choose what to start with—even if you think a different choice would be better.	**Force your child to do the interventions that you prefer** You making all the choices can feel disempowering to kids. If you tell them to try one technique and they really want to do a different one, that is a surefire way to ensure they won't stick with the intervention. Feel free to make suggestions, but allow them to ultimately decide—especially teens.
Try interventions more than once No intervention will free your child from anxiety on the first try. That's not a fair expectation! The anxiety took a long time to develop, and it'll take a long time—and some considerable effort—for it to feel manageable.	**Try an intervention once and declare that it doesn't work** Don't be quick to give up. Instead, be sure to give the interventions a chance to work. Determine a routine with your child for how often they will practice their new coping skills. Be as specific as possible. An example would be asking your child to commit to something like the following: "Every morning after I brush my teeth, I'm going to practice my intervention in my room for five minutes." Reward your child for their efforts and for sticking with the process. This is hard work!

you may want to introduce an intervention immediately—which can't be done if it requires access to supplies or the ability to get to a different setting.

Another reason why one of the interventions should be one that can be done anywhere is because it can be difficult for you to remember

Table 3.2 Getting the Most Out of the Interventions

Do	Don't
Make it fun The more fun the process is, the more likely your child will practice and master the interventions. Try suggesting various interventions as activities for the car or at bedtime. Or present the ideas as a game or experiment.	**Make it a chore** No one wants another boring and tedious chore in their day. End of story.
Be creative about incentives and ways to bond Be creative with ways to spend positive time with your child. Screen time doesn't have to be off the table entirely as an option, but also think about some things that you and your child can do together that involves more interaction.	**Rely solely on screen time as a reward or way to connect** It is tempting to use screen time as a way to spend positive time with your child or to offer it as a reward. But keep in mind that if you use it too frequently it begins to lose its power . . . and then you're back at square one. Additionally, screens do not provide the human connection our nervous systems need, and too much screen time can have adverse effects on physical and mental health.
Know when to call it quits Even though we don't want you to stop doing something before it has a chance to work, we trust that you also know when something just isn't right. Maybe your kid hates doing an intervention, maybe an intervention needs to be tweaked, maybe you need the support of a therapist or parent consultant. If an intervention is not working, modify it so it works better for your child, or try a different one.	**Keep doing what is clearly not working** We give you lots of intervention options for a reason! As we noted in the introduction, this is *not* a one-size-fits-all process. You know your child best, and when an intervention is just not working, pick (or better yet, have your child pick) something else that may be more engaging and, therefore, effective.

specific interventions when your own anxiety is heightened. It may also be the case that your child may be in a new setting that triggers anxiety symptoms. If your child is only prepared to do their go-to intervention in a specific place, they may have a hard time using it when they need it most—in new and stressful situations. Having a technique to address anxiety that can be done in any setting can make life easier for the whole family—your child especially.

Dive in and enjoy! Try to see working with these interventions as a fun activity for you and your child—a bonding experience. Hopefully before you know it, your child will be telling *you* to go to your calm down spot (p. 112) and do some progressive muscle relaxation (p. 109)!

Child Self-Assessment

One of the first steps toward managing anxious feelings is understanding those feelings. Activity 3.1 helps you explore what anxiety means for you. If you are not sure what the answers are to some of these questions, that's okay! Answer the ones you can and come back to any you left blank at a later date. And remember, there is no right or wrong here—it's an opportunity to learn more about yourself!

> **Parent Note:** If you have young children, they will need some help to complete this, but be careful not to sway their answers.

Activity 3.1: Child Activity
Anxiety Self-Reflection

Instructions for children: Complete this form and think about whether you learn anything new about yourself in doing so. If you feel comfortable, share these responses with someone you trust.

1. I feel anxious when I am in this location (like at school or at home or at recess): _____.

2. I feel anxious when I am doing this activity (like when in a social situation, at school, when practicing my instrument): _____

   _____.

3. One thing I want my parents to know about my anxiety is _____

_____.

4. I have had feelings of anxiety since I was _____ years old.

Complete these sentences (there are no right or wrong answers).

5. I wish my anxiety _____

_____.

6. A person I trust to help me with my anxiety is _____

_____.

7. One thing I want my friends to know about my anxiety is _____

_____.

8. The hardest part about my anxiety is _____

_____.

9. A way that I can learn more about my anxiety it to _____

_____.

10. I cope with my anxiety by _____

_____.

11. Something I like about this way of coping is _____

_____.

12. Something I don't like about this way of coping is _____

_____.

13. One thing I want my teachers to know about my anxiety is _____

_____.

14. When my anxiety feels overwhelming, I can tell _____

_____.

(In other words, who do you feel you can turn to when your anxiety gets uncomfortable and you feel you need a little more support?)

15. Other things I want to communicate about my anxiety are _____

_____.

Cognitive Restructuring Interventions and Exercises

Remember: You do not need to try out all of these interventions and exercises.

The goal is to find a few that work well for your child.

Activity 3.2: Cognitive Restructuring Child Activity

Worry Jar

Best for: All ages

Materials: Paper, pen or pencil, jar, and scissors

Instructions for children: This exercise helps you learn to put your anxiety aside, at least temporarily. Consider the anxieties, stresses, or worries that are on your mind. Take a few moments to write down a word or sentence that represents each of the concerns that you feel regularly. Write each concern down on its own piece of paper. Once you have written each concern on the paper, place each paper in the jar. As you put each paper in the jar, tell yourself that you are putting that worry away for now and you don't have to think about it. The worries still exist, but they are safe, in another place (the jar), and away from you. Anytime a new worry or worries pop up that are not already in your jar, get another piece of paper and add the new one(s). Your worry jar can also be used for Activity 3.3, Worry Time, on the next page.

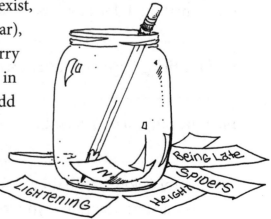

Activity 3.3: Cognitive Restructuring Child Activity

Worry Time

Best for: All ages

Materials: Worry jar (see Activity 3.2), clock, watch, or timer

Instructions for children: Anxiety has an important purpose in our lives, and we don't want to get rid of it. Anxiety can help us stay motivated to finish tasks like homework. It can help us stay energized or get us pumped up for a big game. It can also send us warnings when there is the potential for something scary to happen, like a bee sting. That said, when it feels like you spend too much time every day worrying, it can be disruptive.

This exercise is about being aware of and taking responsibility for the time that you spend worrying. Choose a certain time during your day when you will allow yourself to worry. When that time comes around, set your timer for fifteen minutes, pick a piece of paper out of your worry jar (see Activity 3.2), and spend that time thinking about it. If fifteen minutes seems too long, make your worry time a shorter period. Schedule your

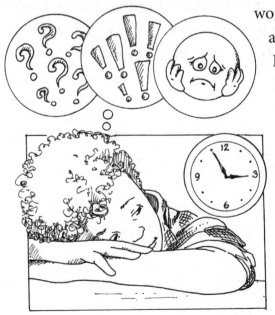

worry time at the same time every day, and think about the best time for you. For example, do not schedule it right before you go to sleep if it will make it hard for you to fall asleep. Or do not schedule it for before school if you are always rushing in the morning to make the bus. If every day feels too often, schedule your worry time less frequently. Concerns will, of course, come to you outside of this set time. When that happens, do your best to let them go by. Remind yourself you'll have time to think about them soon when worry time rolls around again. Sometimes you may find that you don't want to use your worry time for thinking about your worries and it is okay to skip it. You are learning to control your worries instead of allowing your worries to control you.

Activity 3.4: Cognitive Restructuring Child Activity

My Favorite Things

Best for: All ages

Materials: Pen or pencil

Instructions for children: Often people are so busy doing what we *have* to do, we don't take the time to do what we *should* or *want* to do. This is true for everyone—even kids! On this page, make a list of the activities and things that make you feel happy or calm. Focus on those things that really make you feel good or give you energy. Include things on your list that you can do in a variety of locations where you spend time almost every day (like home or school) and that don't cost much money. In other words, don't focus on zip-lining in Mexico or a trip to Walt Disney World! Commit to doing one of the things on your list on a daily, weekly, or monthly basis.

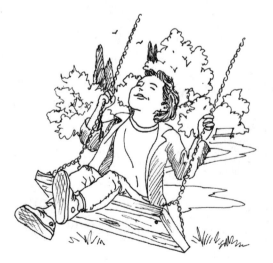

Parent Note: You can do this exercise on behalf of your child if they are too young to write their own list. Ask your child about simple things that you know they enjoy—maybe building with Legos, going for a walk to the park, or spending relaxed time with an extended family member. Try to pick an activity where there is some form of interaction between your child and the adult they are spending time with. Activities like video games and other screen time should be limited.

Some things I can do to treat myself at home are:

1. _____

2. _____

3. _____

Some things I can do to treat myself at school are:

1. _____

2. _____

3. _____

Some things I can do to treat myself for free are:

1. _____

2. _____

3. _____

Some things I can do to treat myself when I'm alone are:

1. _____

2. _____

3. _____

Activity 3.5: Cognitive Restructuring Child Activity

Daily Mood Record

*Samantha's Top Pick

Best for: All ages

Materials: Pen or pencil

Instructions for children: It can be helpful to keep track of and record moods for a number of reasons. For starters, keeping a record can help us understand how our moods may shift or how the patterns in our lives affect our moods. For example, think about how you feel on school days versus on weekends or how you feel on a sunny day versus a rainy day or on a day you have a cold. Having more information about our moods can help us prepare for and manage mood shifts. Additionally, tracking can be a great reminder that things are not always bad and that daily life is almost never all good or all bad. Our brains tend to remember difficulties more easily than successes. By keeping a daily log of your mood, you train yourself to remember the positive things that happen and to keep in mind that a lot of time things are actually going well.

Periodically, look back at your daily logs to consider your moods over a given period of time. Identify any patterns and ask yourself what may be the cause of regular or common ups and downs. This is a good time to remind yourself that things change, so even if you are experiencing challenges now, there is always opportunity for things to get better. Tell yourself that *all things—even difficult things—eventually pass*, so you will not have these feelings forever. It can be helpful to remind yourself that later today or by early next week, this feeling may no longer be with you.

Here we've created a sample log for you to try, but there are lots of ways to log your moods. For example, you can put a smiley or frowny face on the days of a wall or desk calendar to record your mood for each day. Or you can keep a more in-depth journal about what happened during each day and how you felt about it. And there are many mood-tracking apps for smartphones if you prefer to keep your mood diary electronically. It's also helpful to pay close attention to changes in your sleep schedule.

Parent Note: For young children, ask them about their feelings, but also use some of their own assessment when logging moods.

How do I feel today? Circle an emoticon (or two) and write an explanation.

Sample entry: Wednesday 😃 😐 😧 😨 😴 😠 A reason I feel this today is: *I'm tired because I had bad dreams last night and didn't sleep well and then I didn't have time to watch my favorite show this morning. Then at recess it rained and we didn't get to go outside.*

Monday 😃 😐 😧 😨 😴 😠 A reason I feel this today is:

_____

Tuesday 😃 😐 😧 😨 😴 😠 A reason I feel this today is:

_____

Wednesday 😃 😐 😧 😨 😴 😠 A reason I feel this today is:

_____

Thursday 😃 😐 😧 😨 😴 😠 A reason I feel this today is:

_____

Friday 😃 😐 😧 😨 😴 😠 A reason I feel this today is:

_____

Saturday 😃 😐 😧 😨 😴 😠 A reason I feel this today is:

_____

Sunday 😃 😐 😧 😨 😴 😠 A reason I feel this today is:

_____

Activity 3.6: Cognitive Restructuring Child Activity

Self-Talk Cheerleader!

Best for: All ages

Materials: Pen or pencil

Instructions for children: Self-talk is the things we tell ourselves throughout the course of the day. Sometimes we are very aware of these things and other times they seem to come into our minds without us even realizing. Either way, self-talk can have a big impact on self-confidence and overall mood. If you are always telling yourself you are going to do a bad job at something or that you are not smart, not funny, or not likeable, you may start to believe it. It may impact your willingness to try things or your confidence in group situations. This can ultimately impact your mood and create a sense of anxiety and sadness. If your self-talk is kind and compassionate, the way you may talk to a good friend—honest, yet always kind—it can feel like encouragement and support.

Take a look at the statements below. In the line below each statement, write a response that you may give to someone you care about if they were to make statements like these.

After you have gone through the practice statements, think about how you turn your own concerns into negative self-talk. Think about how you could give yourself a pep talk instead. You can talk to yourself in your mind or you can speak out loud and that's totally fine too. The idea is to acknowledge your strengths and remind yourself that you are strong and you can get through whatever stressors lie ahead.

Your friend says: My mom and dad probably hate me because I never clean up my room.

Your response: No way! Your mom and dad love you so much. Think of all the things they do for you and all the fun times you have together. It's just a parent's job to remind us to clean up and stuff.

Your friend says: I'm never the one who scores the goals at the soccer games.

Your response: I've seen you at the games and you always provide the assist. Without you, your teammate wouldn't score!

Now think of some of your own examples:

Your thoughts: _____

_____

_____

_____

Your self pep talk: _____

_____

_____

_____

Your thoughts: _____

_____

_____

_____

Your self pep talk: _____

_____

_____

_____

Activity 3.7: Cognitive Restructuring Child Activity

Journal of Joy

Best for: All ages

Materials: Pen or pencil and notebook or journal

Instructions for children: Journaling is a great way to reflect on and express our feelings. Sometimes journaling can help people get in touch with feelings they didn't even know they had. However, not everyone loves to write long journal entries about their concerns and fears. So, in this exercise you journal only about positive moments, experiences, and events. Take a moment to reflect on your day and note the moments that stand out to you as being the best. Make journal entries about these positive moments. Write descriptions, make drawings, compose poetry, or jot down lists. Think especially about simple joys and pleasure. For example, joyous things may include sunshine, a quick playful moment with a friend, or a sweet, juicy orange you ate at lunch.

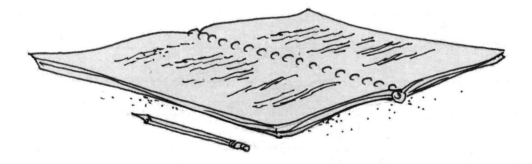

Activity 3.8: Cognitive Restructuring Child Activity

Get-Over-The-Fear Goals

Best for: All ages

Materials: Paper and pen or pencil

Instructions for children: A goal is something you are hoping to achieve or working toward. It may be very short-term, like scoring in tomorrow's hockey game, or longer term, like going to college someday. Goals are most likely to be achieved if they are concrete, stated, and measurable. *Concrete* means a goal is clear and specific—think "I want to get three As this term" rather than "I want to do better." *Stated* is just what it sounds like—you have to say the goal. Keeping the idea as something that loosely floats around your mind is less likely to result in change than actually saying it out loud or writing it down. And *measurable* means that there is a way to know, or measure, if you have actually achieved the goal you set. If you say "I want to be more independent," it is more difficult to measure whether you have accomplished it than "I want to pack my lunch for school three days each week."

It also helps to break goals down into small pieces that can be managed one step at a time. With the example above of aiming to get three As, you may want to set some mini goals that help you work toward it. You may say, "I need to do my homework every night and study for one hour the day before every test in order to work toward the goal of getting three As."

For many people with anxiety, getting over their fears is a goal. In this version of goal setting, you learn to challenge specific fears. This can be done in list form. You can ask for your parents' help if you need it. Start by thinking and talking about fears that you would like to overcome. Once you have identified a fear that troubles you and makes you anxious, name that fear and write it at the top of the paper. Under the fear, list several steps you can take to work toward overcoming it. Anytime you accomplish one of the steps, acknowledge your accomplishment! Give yourself a sticker, cross the step off your list with a big red marker, or share the news with a grown-up or friend.

Examples of fears, goals, and small steps

Fear: Spiders   The Pool   Talking to Grown-Ups
Goals:

Get over my fear of spiders	Be able to swim in the pool this summer	Be less nervous when talking to adults

Steps to Reach My Goals:

1. Read a book about spiders.	1. Visit a local pool.	1. Wave at adults I know when I see them.
2. Look at pictures of spiders online or in a book.	2. Put my toes in the pool.	2. Say hello to my teachers at the beginning of class.
3. Hold a cup with a spider in it.	3. Put my legs in the pool.	3. Raise my hand when I know the answer in class.
	4. Go in the water up to my waist.	

Your turn! List your fears, your goals, and the steps you can take to get over your fears and achieve your goals!

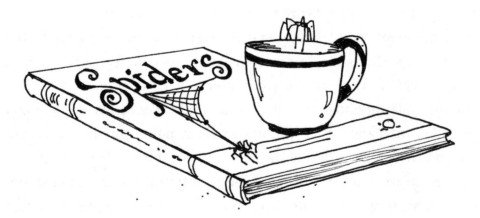

My Fear:_____

My Goal:_____

Steps to Reach My Get-Over-The-Fear Goal:

Step 1: _____

_____

Step 2: _____

_____

Step 3: _____

_____

My Fear:_____

My Goal:_____

Steps to Reach My Get-Over-The-Fear Goal:

Step 1: _____

_____

Step 2: _____

_____

Step 3: _____

_____

My Fear:_____

My Goal:_____

Steps to Reach My Get-Over-The-Fear Goal:

Step 1: _____

_____

Step 2: _____

_____

Step 3: _____

_____

Activity 3.9: Cognitive Restructuring Child Activity*

Magic Lego Connection

Best for: Toddlers and preschoolers (Note that unlike most of the other activities in this section, this one is parent-directed.)

Materials: 2+ matching Lego bricks or pennies, pebbles, or any other item small enough to be kept in a pocket (maybe more)

Instructions for parents: This is a helpful tool for separation anxiety, but it can also be tailored to help with certain fears and phobias. Find the same color and size Legos for every member of your family. (This activity can also be done with pennies, pebbles, or any other item small enough to be kept in a pocket.) Tell your child that while you are apart, everyone will have these items in their pockets and that they have to stay in the pocket. Every time your child feels sad, scared, or lonely, they can touch or even just think about the item and it will send a little "zap" of energy to the items in the pockets of all their family members. Parents can explain to their child that the item is not magic on its own but that the connection that it creates makes it magical for your family. Remember to keep the magical thinking going by asking about it once you're all back together. And don't forget to "recharge" the items overnight!

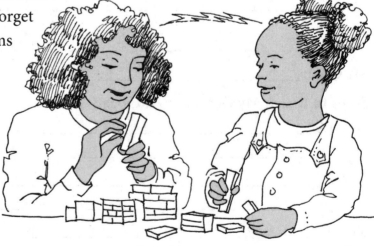

---

*Suggested for battling separation anxiety

Activity 3.10: Cognitive Restructuring Child Activity*

Watch the Clock

Best for: Toddlers and preschoolers (Note that unlike most of the other activities in this section, this one is parent-directed.)

Materials: Clock or watch

Instructions for parents: This exercise is especially helpful for children who experience separation anxiety. Buy your child a small digital clock or watch and teach them about how the first number (the hour indicator) represents a time of day. You may even want to cover up the second two numbers so that only the first is visible. Tell your child what number they will see when it is time for you to return, and be sure to be on time! (If your return time is typically 5:45 p.m., you would want to tell your child that you will be home by the time it gets to 6 rather than when it turns to 5 to avoid them waiting an extended period.) This intervention usually needs to be used only for a short period of time—once kids start to know and trust that you will be back, they feel less and less need for the clock.

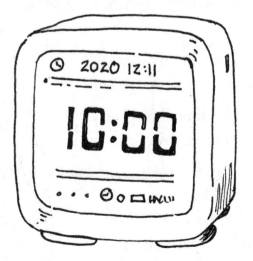

---

*Great for kids with separation anxiety

Activity 3.11: Cognitive Restructuring Child Activity

Four Quick Questions

Best for: Grade-school kids, tweens, and teens

Materials: None needed

Instructions for children: This intervention helps you explore and better understand your anxious thoughts. The goal is to think about how realistic your anxious thoughts are. Often our thoughts and feelings make something seem worse than it really is. By examining our thoughts, we often realize that things are not as bad as we imagine them to be. This will help you recognize that you have power over the way you react to these thoughts and feelings. It is also helpful to recognize that feelings are not facts. This means that just because you feel something, that does not mean it is true. For example, just because you think no one will talk to you at the birthday party you are attending does not make it true! You could end up going, meet some new friends, and have a great time. This exercise provides a way for you to examine the truth of your thoughts and feelings.

When you have an anxious negative thought, ask yourself these four questions about it:

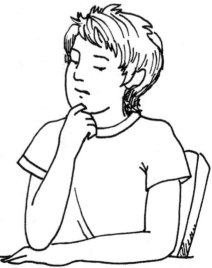

1. Is this thought causing my anxiety to feel better or worse?

2. Where did I learn this thought? (Can I remember the first time I had this thought?)

3. Is this thought logical and reasonable? (Is it something that has ever happened or could really happen?)

4. Is this thought true? (Is there evidence for it or is it just a feeling I have?)

Here are a couple of examples of how this may go:

Thought:

Dogs are scary and dangerous and I worry that one will bite me.

1. Is this thought causing my anxiety to feel better or worse?

   Worse.

2. Where did I learn this thought?

   I've never liked dogs, but I can't remember a specific time or reason it started.

3. Is this thought logical and reasonable?

   Yes, sometimes dogs are aggressive and may bite people, but I have never known anyone who got bit and it isn't very common. Actually, I know a lot of people who have dogs, and most of them are gentle and playful.

4. Is this thought true?

   Thinking through this makes me think maybe it is more of a feeling than a fact that dogs are scary.

Thought:

I failed an English test and I'll probably never get into the college I wanted to go to.

1. Is this thought causing my anxiety to feel better or worse?

   Worse.

2. Where did I learn this thought?

   Teachers and friends keep saying that you really need perfect grades to be accepted at that school. I've known that since middle school.

3. Is this thought logical and reasonable?

Yes, they have a lot of great candidates—why would they ever take me when they can take someone who has perfect grades? But I guess they do talk about how important it is to be well rounded, and I have great grades overall and this was only one test, not even my final grade.

4. Is this thought true?

The truth is that my dream college has an average required GPA and I will still fall in that range. Maybe this is just a feeling.

If this exercise is helpful for you, write the four questions on an index card or scrap of paper and keep the list with you so that it's available whenever you need it. When you feel an anxious thought getting out of control, ask yourself the four questions and take comfort in your answers.

Activity 3.12: Cognitive Restructuring Child Activity

The Three Cs

Best for: Grade-school kids, tweens, and teens

Materials: None needed

Instructions for children: The three Cs can help you change negative thoughts and thought patterns. Use it whenever you remember to, but try to do it at least once per week. Notice when you find it helpful so you can use it again in those types of situations. The three Cs stand for Catch, Check, and Challenge.

Catch It ➡ Check It ➡ Challenge It

Catch your worrisome thoughts, whether they zoom by in your mind like a car or drift by more slowly like clouds in the sky. No matter what speed your current concern is moving, catch it. You can catch your worry by writing it down, saying it out loud, or telling a friend or family member about it. By doing this, you make the worrisome thought more real—you have caught it. Remember, it's your thought, and you may have more control over it than you think.

Check in with yourself about whether this worry is even true. Do some fact checking! Is there evidence for your fear, or is it just a feeling you have? Remember, *feelings are not facts!* (By the way, this statement—*feelings are not facts*—can be helpful to keep in mind and repeat to yourself, silently or out loud.)

Challenge your thoughts. Create a character for your worry and talk to it or "fight" it off. Perhaps your worry is a green blob and you can smush it or tear it up to make it smaller. If you are having trouble coming up with a character, books are great tools to develop these. Some of the books we have listed in the resource chapter (p. 150–153) would work well for this, including *David and the Worry Beast*, *Hey Warrior*, and *Is a Worry Worrying You?* Let the thought know that you're pushing back on it and aren't going to stand for it.

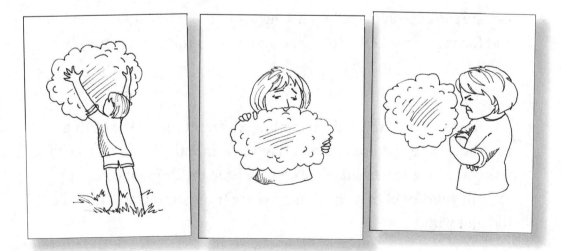

Activity 3.13: Cognitive Restructuring Child Activity

ACT (Acknowledge, Consider, Try)

Best for: Grade-school kids, tweens, and teens

Materials: None needed

Instructions for children: ACT stands for Acknowledge, Consider, Try. ACT allows you to acknowledge the unhelpful thoughts that you have, question those thoughts, and do something different instead. Although there are thoughts that automatically pop into your head, you don't always have to agree with them! Automatic doesn't mean true. Challenge your thoughts with this exercise.

When you find yourself having a negative or uncomfortable thought, such as thinking that your teacher doesn't like you, take these three steps:

1. *Acknowledge the thought*

   Acknowledging the thought means recognizing it's there and that it's not helpful or comfortable.

2. *Consider*

   Considering involves really thinking about the thought for a moment and focusing on whether it is true and/or why the thought may be there.

3. *Try*

   The final step is to try to do something different instead of having this thought repeat itself in your day/week/month. Try to replace this thought with an alternative idea. Every time the thought comes up, remind yourself of the new thing you are trying to replace the old thought with.

Example:

Thought:

My teacher is never going to like me or think I'm smart.

Acknowledge the thought:

My thought is that the teacher doesn't like me or think I am smart.

Consider:

What has my teacher done or said that makes me think this is true? Is it possible I just made this up because I am nervous around her? Has she ever said anything to support this thought?

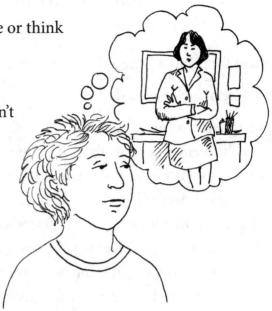

Try:

Try out an alternate thought such as, "I'm going to try and tell myself that she is just being firm because it's the beginning of the school year," or, "I feel good about how hard I'm working and I hope my teacher notices. But if she doesn't, I can still feel good and proud about working hard."

Activity 3.14: Cognitive Restructuring Child Activity

Reframing

Melissa's Top Pick

Best for: Grade-school kids, tweens, and teens

Materials: None needed

Instructions for children: Reframing challenges you to look at something in a different way or from a different perspective. Have you ever seen a picture in one frame and then when the picture is in a different frame, it has a totally different look? Sometimes even a different feeling? That is what you're aiming for here. By imagining the way someone else would think of the same idea you have in your head, you are giving it a different picture frame, thereby changing the look and feel.

In this activity, we list a few examples of things people worry about (tests, storms, flying). Pretend the first thought in each group is your worry and then challenge yourself to think of how someone else may be thinking about the same thing. When you do this, it is "reframing."

After thinking through the examples, consider a worry or problem that has been on your mind recently. Now imagine somebody else thinking about this same worry and how it may look from their point of view.

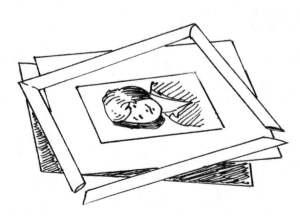
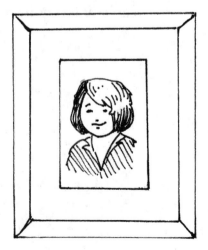

Your thought:

I did terribly on that test. I've always known I'm bad at math. I'm going to fail that class.

Consider a reframe:

For help, consider what your teacher's thought might be about how you did on that test. Or what your friend might say to you if they knew you did poorly on your test. Their perspectives may help you to develop your own reframe.

Your thought:

The sky looks dark and I'm afraid there may be a storm. I'll have to walk home in the thunder and lightning.

Consider a reframe:

For help, consider how a farmer or an ecologist thinks about a rainstorm. Is there anything about this that could be silly or adventurous?

Your thought:

I don't want to go on that airplane. It could crash!

Consider a reframe:

For help, consider how pilots and flight attendants think about flying. How do they feel safe flying all the time? _____

_____

Your thought: (write down something you are worrying about lately)

_____

_____

_____

What are some ways I can challenge myself to look at this differently? How might someone else see this differently?

Activity 3.15: Cognitive Restructuring Child Activity

Hit the Snooze Button

Best for: Grade-school kids, tweens, and teens

Materials: None needed

Instructions for children: When people sense danger, the fear center in our brains, which is called the amygdala, gets activated and sounds its alarms. This is known as the fight, flight, or freeze response. Fight, flight, or freeze is a protective factor that keeps us safe in times of real danger. (See chapter 1, p. 12, and appendix A, "Understanding Anxiety-Related Structures and Processes.") But for people with anxiety, the alarms often go off even when there is no actual threat.

Sometimes, if you can catch yourself in time, you can let yourself know that there is no need to be alarmed and you can avoid activating your fight, flight, or freeze response. We call this hitting the snooze button. You hear the alarm go off, but you shut it down before it rings too long. By hitting the button, you let your response know to come back later. In this case, the "later" is when there is an actual threat. As you get more in touch with your anxiety, you will start to notice things that happen in your body and in your mind just as your anxiety is kicking in.

These reactions look different in different people but generally present exactly how they sound. Fight is a rush of energy creating the feeling of a need to react. Flight is a rush of energy creating the need to run or escape. Freeze is a flooding of thoughts and feelings that result in an inability to move. Think about how people respond when a bee lands on them. One person may try and hit the bee (fight), another may try and run from it (flight), and one may stand as still as can be (freeze).

Recognizing these signs and telling yourself "I'm hitting snooze" may be enough of a distraction and change of course to prevent activating your fight, flight, or freeze response when it's not necessary. You can hit the snooze by writing the words "I'm hitting snooze," making a note in your phone, or telling a person close to you that you are hitting the snooze button. You can also just repeat "I'm hitting snooze" quietly to yourself or silently in your head. These techniques can be combined with other calming activities such as Body Scan (p. 108), Stress Balls (p. 116), or Create Your Own Mantra (p. 128) to make them feel even more powerful.

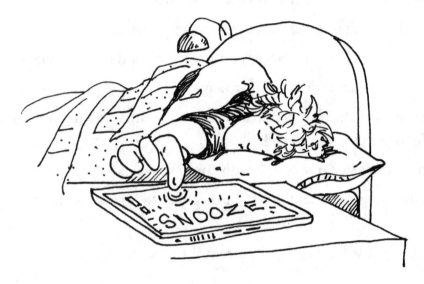

Activity 3.16: Cognitive Restructuring Child Activity

Change Your Vocabulary!

Best for: Grade-school kids, tweens, and teens

Materials: Pen or pencil

Instructions for children: Overgeneralizations and all-or-nothing statements—like when we use the words "always" or "never"—are two ways that language can contribute to anxious feelings. We list some examples of each of these below. In this exercise, we encourage you to notice when you are using these types of statements and challenge yourself to find alternatives.

You may want to create a bucket of alternative synonyms (different words that mean the same thing) or phrases that you can pick from when you're struggling.

Parent Note: Help younger children by pointing out and suggesting changes to their language when they use these types of expressions.

Overgeneralization: I am *always* so awkward.

Alternative: I felt awkward on the first day at my new school.

Overgeneralization: I am *never* going to be a good baseball player.

Alternative: I had a rough game today.

All-or-nothing statement: If I can't do well on this spelling test, I'll *never* be able to pass the third grade.

Alternative: It's just one test, it won't hold me back.

All-or-nothing statement: *Everyone* is going to be mad at me if I miss this goal.

Alternative: It will be a huge bummer if I miss this goal.

Instead of . . .	Use . . .
"I can't . . ."	"This is difficult . . ."
"I'll never . . ."	"This will take practice . . ."
"This is always . . ."	"In this case or example, it is . . ."

Some unhelpful words I use are:

Some more productive language I can try is:

_____   _____

_____   _____

_____   _____

_____   _____

_____   _____

Activity 3.17: Cognitive Restructuring Child Activity*

Checked It Checklist

Best for: Grade-school kids, tweens, and teens

Materials: Pen or pencil, notebook, and clock or watch

Instructions for children: When some people become anxious, they may think the same concerning thought over and over. This is called a rumination or an obsessive thought. In an effort to get rid of these kinds of uncomfortable thoughts, sometimes people try to calm them by taking action. This is a compulsion, and it can become a problem. For example, you can't stop thinking that you forgot to lock your front door, and the only way you can get relief from that thought is to repeatedly check that the door is locked. Perhaps even after you leave for school and you have double-checked and know the door is locked, you still are bothered by the same desire to go home and check again a few hours later. As you can see, this sort of behavior can be disruptive.

If you struggle with this type of obsessive thought and compulsive behavior pattern, try making a checklist for yourself. Write down the thought you have and the behavior you typically do to soothe it. Every time you do the behavior, record the time you did it in the notebook. Every time you think about the behavior but don't do it, put a star in the time column. This can help you to remember that the real concern has been addressed. This helps because, when you look at your record, you can see that you already did the behavior, and your written note is there to remind you of that. As you become aware of your behavior, you may be less inclined to think about it so frequently. This can help stop intrusive thoughts from creeping into your mind too frequently.

---

*Great for kids who struggle with repetitive thoughts or for those with diagnosed obsessive compulsive tendencies

Thought	Behavior	Time
_____	_____	_____
_____	_____	

Thought	Behavior	Time
_____	_____	_____
_____	_____	

Thought	Behavior	Time
_____	_____	_____
_____	_____	

Activity 3.18: Cognitive Restructuring Child Activity

Plan for the "Problem"

Best for: Grade-school kids, tweens, and teens

Materials: Pen or pencil

Instructions for children: Some worrisome thoughts are based on future concerns that, in many cases, never actually happen. If you find yourself thinking a lot of "what if" type thoughts (*what if* my friend is mad at me, *what if* I fail that test, *what if* I lose the race), we encourage you to think about the concern and make a plan for addressing it. Although there are exceptions, typically if you can't plan a response to a worry, it's not actually a problem. At least not yet.

Choose a "what if" concern of your own. Then think through the following questions to determine if the problem is one that you need to be stressing about right now.

Example:

My worry is: What if I trip and fall during opening night of the school musical?

1. Is there anything I can do *in this moment* to make this problem go away? If there is, these are the things I can do to feel better: *I can practice the harder steps right now and each day. I can also remind myself that one person fell during last year's musical and it really wasn't a big deal.*

2. Is there anything else I can do *today* to make this problem go away? If there is, these are the things I can do today to make this worry go away: *I can't make it go away completely. But I can call my costar and see if they want to practice some of the more tricky moves with me.*

3. Is there anything else I can do to make myself feel better about this worry? If there is, these are the things I can do to feel better about this worry: *One last thing I can do is talk to the other kids in the play about my worries—they might have some good advice.*

My worry is: What if _____

_____

_____

_____

1. Is there anything I can do in this moment to make this problem go away? If there is, these are the things I can do in this moment to make this fear go away: _____

_____

_____

_____

2. Is there anything I can do today to make this problem go away? If there is, these are the things I can do today to make this worry go away: _____

_____

_____

_____

3. Is there anything else I can do to make myself feel better about this worry? If there is, these are the things I can do to feel better about this worry:

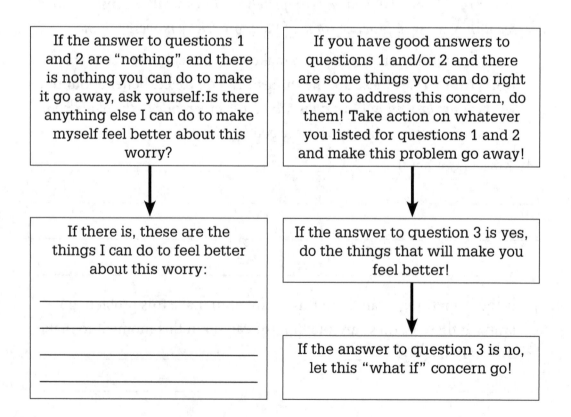

If the answer to questions 1 and 2 are "nothing" and there is nothing you can do to make it go away, ask yourself:Is there anything else I can do to make myself feel better about this worry?

If you have good answers to questions 1 and/or 2 and there are some things you can do right away to address this concern, do them! Take action on whatever you listed for questions 1 and 2 and make this problem go away!

If there is, these are the things I can do to feel better about this worry:

_____

_____

_____

_____

If the answer to question 3 is yes, do the things that will make you feel better!

If the answer to question 3 is no, let this "what if" concern go!

For example, if you auditioned for a school play and you are worrying about whether you got the part you wanted, there may be nothing you can do! The worrying isn't helping or changing the situation, and you can't plan to do anything about it because you simply don't yet know if there is something to worry about!

If you can't make a plan to address the problem, it's likely not yet a problem.

Activity 3.19: Cognitive Restructuring Child Activity

The "So What?" Game

Best for: Grade-school kids, tweens, and teens

Materials: Pen or pencil

Instructions for children: Sometimes worries and fears feel bigger and scarier in our minds than they are in real life. In this exercise we ask you to think about some of the things you are concerned about or things you are scared of and imagine what would happen if they actually occurred. Once you start to think your worries and fears through, you may find that you can actually handle them better than you are giving yourself credit for. And you may find they are not as bad as you initially thought. By asking yourself "So what?" you are challenging yourself to think through all the possible outcomes and determine whether they are realistic and manageable. Follow the directions to play this mind game that you can do anytime and anywhere.

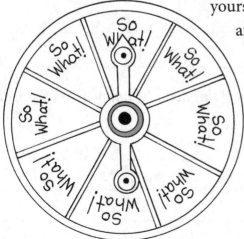

Parent Note: For younger children, help by prompting them with "so what then" questions as they navigate the worry in their mind. Oftentimes young children may name a fear that is not likely or is absolutely impossible. It is okay to gently explain why that part of the fear is not probable.

Here is an example for doing this exercise with a young child. If your child says, "What if at school I get locked in the bathroom?" you may say, "That would be scary. So what would you do if that happened?" They may say that they'd feel scared or cry or yell. You can continue with, "Yes, I can see why you'd do that. So what if you did cry or yell or feel scared?" If your child responds, "Then my friends would know," you may say, "Yes, your friends would know, and so what if that happens?" They may say, "I would feel embarrassed," and you may say, "So what then?" At some point your child will hopefully get to a place where the outcome doesn't seem all that bad or they recognize the outcome may be uncomfortable but not unbearable.

Step 1: Write down what you are worried about.

The thing I am worried about is: _____

_____

_____

_____

Step 2: Ask yourself, "So what?" *So what if this actually happens? What will that be like? What will it mean?*

If this actually happens it will be like this: _____

_____

_____

_____

Step 3: Continue to ask yourself the question from step 2 until you have addressed all the reasons it feels scary.

These things could also happen if this thing occurs: _____

_____

_____

Activity 3.20: Cognitive Restructuring Child Activity

SUDS

Best for: Tweens and teens

Materials: Pen or pencil

Instructions for children: SUDS stands for Subjective Units of Distress Scale. This scale is used to measure the level of distress a person experiences in a given situation. It's almost like an anxiety thermometer! In this exercise you learn to measure your anxiety in different situations. This will help you learn more about your personal relationship with anxiety and give you a chance to better manage it.

Here is an abbreviated version of the traditional SUDS scale:

10	I am at my highest level of anxiety. I'm feeling the worst possible anxiety I could imagine.
8–9	I am very anxious and it is starting to feel intolerable. I'm having trouble focusing.
6–7	I am very aware of my anxiety and it feels very unpleasant but is manageable.
5	I feel some anxiety but it is tolerable.
3–4	I feel a slight amount of tension/ mild distress but I am able to focus.
1–2	I feel minimal to no anxiety or tension.
0	I am totally and completely relaxed.

Use the space below or a journal to track your SUDS score in both routine, unexciting situations and anxiety-provoking experiences. Doing this will help you identify patterns in how your anxiety affects you. Once you see patterns, you can work to develop coping strategies to get you through times when you have high SUDS scores. You can use some of the other intervention activities in this workbook to help reduce your anxiety during these times—the mindfulness activities (pp. 99–112) are a great place to start.

Score	Date/Time	What's happening/on my mind?
Score	Date/Time	What's happening/on my mind?
Score	Date/Time	What's happening/on my mind?
Score	Date/Time	What's happening/on my mind?
Score	Date/Time	What's happening/on my mind?

My SUDS score is highest when:

_____

_____

_____

_____

_____

My SUDS score is lowest when:

_____

_____

_____

_____

_____

Activity 3.21: Cognitive Restructuring Child Activity*

Self-Evaluation

Best for: Tweens and teens

Materials: None needed

Instructions for children: Self-talk refers to the things we tell ourselves or the way we speak to ourselves during the day. Sometimes we are aware of self-talk and other times self-talk comes into our minds without us even realizing it. Self-talk can have an impact on our self-confidence and overall mood. If your self-talk is positive, such as, "I am going rock my first day of my new job," it can build up your self-esteem; if it is negative, such as, "Why do I always make so many mistakes?" it can make you feel worse about yourself. This exercise will help you identify the negative things you say to yourself regularly.

_____

*Great for kids with low self-esteem

Review the things you say as part of your self-talk. The next time you find yourself saying something negative to yourself, ask yourself the following questions:

❖ What's happening in this moment?

❖ What am I telling myself about this situation?

❖ Am I putting myself down?

❖ Am I being self-critical?

Follow up with these questions:

❖ Are the things I am thinking (my thoughts) facts or opinions?

❖ Is it helpful when I think about myself and my situation in this way?

❖ Are there other ways I can look at this situation? How would a friend, parent, or teacher see it? (Also see Activity 3.14, Reframing.)

❖ What are the positive things I could be telling myself?

❖ What would be a more helpful way for me to think about myself and this situation?

Example:

Self-Talk: No one at school likes me. I'm never funny and I don't have anything interesting to add to any group conversation.

❖ What's happening in this moment? *I'm feeling left out and sad.*

❖ What am I telling myself about this situation? *That no one likes me and I have no friends.*

❖ Am I putting myself down? *Yes.*

❖ Am I being self-critical? *Yes.*

❖ Are the things I am thinking (my thoughts) facts or opinions? *Opinions.*

❖ Is it helpful when I think about myself and my situation in this way? *No.*

❖ Are there other ways I can look at this situation? How would a friend, parent, or teacher see this situation? (Also see Activity 3.14, Reframing.) *I'm a little quieter than many of my friends, but I have always been included.*

❖ What are the positive things I could be telling myself? *I'm thoughtful and not someone who talks just to talk, but I love listening to others.*

❖ What would be a more helpful way for me to think about myself and this situation? *I add some balance to our friend group.*

Review your answers. What do you notice about them? Do you see any patterns in the way you are talking negatively to yourself? Would you ever speak this way to your friends or allow them to speak about themselves this way? Question why you are so hard on yourself and what you may want to tell yourself instead.

Mindfulness Interventions and Exercises

Remember: You do not need to try out all of these interventions and exercises.

The goal is to find a few that work well for your child.

Activity 3.22: Mindfulness Child Activity
Deep Breathing Basics

Best for: All ages

Materials: None needed

Instructions for children: Deep breathing is one of the best ways to reduce stress. It works because breathing sends oxygen to the brain, which stimulates the part of the brain (the parasympathetic nervous system) that helps the body relax after essential functions like eating (see appendix A,

"Understanding Anxiety-Related Structures and Processes"). This makes us feel calmer.

Lie down or sit comfortably in a chair. Close your eyes and focus on your breath. Take a deep breath in through your nose while counting slowly in your head to three. Gently hold the breath for three seconds. Then push your breath out through your mouth while counting to three. Try to focus only on your breath. Even though it may be hard, try not to think about ordinary things like what you are having for lunch or the chores you need to do. Turn your attention to the breath that is coming in and out of your body. Once you get the hang of deep breathing, you can practice it at any time, in any place. If you want to keep what you are doing private, you can even keep your eyes open. The more you practice, the more normal and natural deep breathing will feel. Then, the easier it will be to use deep breathing as a quick tool for when you are stressed or anxious.

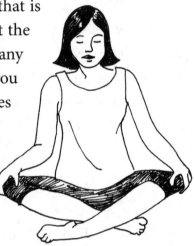

Activity 3.23: Mindfulness Child Activity

Mindful Awareness

Best for: All ages

Materials: None needed

Instructions for children: When we are anxious, we worry about what might happen in the future. This exercise teaches how to bring focus away from future possibilities and back to the present here and now. It can be practiced at any time, in any place.

Wherever you are, take notice of what is around you. Allow yourself to breathe deeply (you may want to combine this exercise with Activity 3.22,

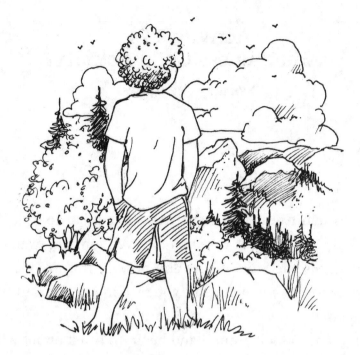

Deep Breathing Basics, p. 99) and think about the pleasant things you notice. (For example, pay attention to the birds chirping, the sun shining, your friend laughing, etc.) Your thoughts may shift to other things—to worries or thoughts about the future or something that happened earlier in the day. Accept that this is happening and then gently bring your awareness back to the current moment.

If you like this exercise, consider taking a mindfulness walk. Take a walk without your phone, without listening to music or speaking. Just simply notice what is around you as you walk.

Parent Note: If doing this with a small child, explain to them that the two of you are taking some moments of quiet time to see what you can notice around you. After a few moments (or when they begin talking), have a conversation about what they experienced.

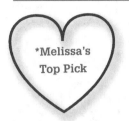

*Melissa's
Top Pick*

Activity 3.24:
Mindfulness Child Activity

Sensory Awareness

*Samantha's
Top Pick*

Best for: All ages

Materials: None needed

Instructions for children: This activity is very similar to Mindful Awareness (see Activity 3.23, p. 100). Like that intervention, this exercise involves bringing your focus back to the here and now. In this exercise, instead of noticing what's around you generally, you're going to pay particular attention to your senses.

Take a moment to look around and begin to think about what each of your five senses (sight, sound, touch, taste, smell) are experiencing. Ask yourself the following questions:

1. What do I see right now? (For example, people walking on the sidewalk, the sun shining, houses, flowers, birds, etc.)

2. What can I hear right now? (For example, my family talking, a truck rumbling down the street, kids laughing, birds singing, etc.)

3. What textures and sensations do I feel right now? (For example, the soft wind, the warm sun, my hair on my shoulders, my backpack on my back, the hard sidewalk under my feet, etc.)

4. What taste do I notice in my mouth? (For example, the mint from my toothpaste, the taste of my gum, etc.)

5. What scents do I smell? (For example, the roses in the neighbor's garden, the lotion I put on this morning, food from the school cafeteria, etc.)

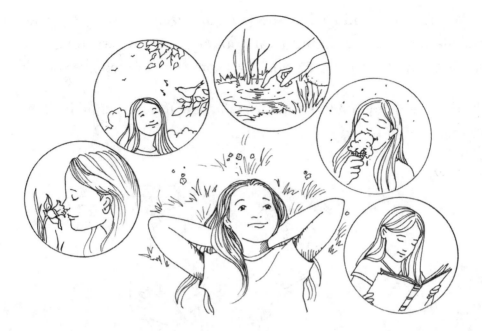

Just like with mindful awareness, sensory awareness can be done at any time and in any place.

Parent Note: If doing this with a small child, walk them through their senses. Pause after explaining each sense to give your child a chance to notice and tell you what they are aware of.

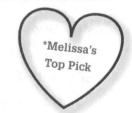

Activity 3.25: Mindfulness Child Activity

Count Five Sounds

*Melissa's Top Pick

Best for: All ages

Materials: None needed

Instructions for children: This activity builds on Activity 3.23, Mindful Awareness (p. 100). It also helps you to bring focus back to the here and now. Take in a few deep breaths and focus on the sounds you notice around you. You may hear things like the washing machine, a person laughing, music playing, a fan humming, a car honking, tree leaves rustling, or a dog barking. Continue to pay attention until you have counted five sounds.

> **Parent Note:** If doing this with a small child, have the child list the sounds they hear and count with them.

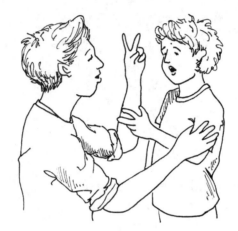

Activity 3.26: Mindfulness Child Activity*

Grounding

Best for: All ages

Materials: None needed

Instructions for children: Grounding helps when you experience anxious feelings. It can be an especially important tool when your anxious feelings are intense and overwhelming. It is especially good in the early stages of panic. Grounding helps you recognize what is actually happening at the present moment, as opposed to what you *feel* might happen in the near future.

Start by closing your eyes. Notice your feet on the ground. Tell yourself (out loud or in your mind) where you are and that you see your feet placed

---

*Great for kids who experience panic

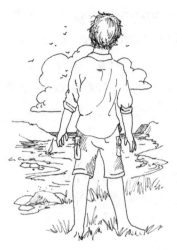

firmly on the ground. Now open your eyes. Look around and note all the things you see in front of you, giving quiet attention to everything you notice. For example, you may notice the pattern of a rug on the floor, a picture on the wall, the tree you can see through a window. Bring all of your awareness and focus to the present moment. As your mind wanders to the future or the past, accept this shift, and then gently bring your awareness back to the current time and place.

Activity 3.27: Mindfulness Child Activity

Visualization

Best for: All ages

Materials: None needed

Instructions for children: Visualization helps you to relax your mind and your body. When you visualize, you close your eyes and vividly imagine a place that is more calming than where you currently are. This exercise can be done alone or with assistance. If you want to do your own visualization, put on some relaxing music and imagine yourself in a favorite place or a place you someday hope to go. Try to imagine how you feel when you are there and enjoy the time you are spending in your imagination. If you would like to try guided visualization, there are many books with visualization scripts. There are also online sites and apps dedicated to guided visualizations and meditations. Experiment with different content and voices. Some people do better with different narrators and different descriptions. Several options are listed in the resources sections of this book (see chapter 5, "Resources," and appendix B, "Additional Support and Professional Treatment Options").

Activity 3.28: Mindfulness Child Activity

Your Happy Place

Best for: All ages

Materials: None needed

Instructions for children: This visualization exercise helps you bring positive feelings and experiences into the current moment by having you create your own happy place. Your personal happy place may be a combination of some favorite places you've been or it may be completely new and made up. Go through each one of your five senses (sight, sound, touch, taste, smell) and think about your experiences in this place and how it affects each sense. Think about your favorite scenery and place yourself there. Then think about what you smell, hear, feel, and taste in your happy place. Make sure to give yourself a few minutes to really imagine and experience each sense. Once you are done with the exercise, remind yourself that you can revisit this place in your mind anytime you'd like.

Now draw what each of your senses experienced in this place. You do not need to be an artist to do this—no one will be judging your work! If you don't enjoy the drawing part of this exercise, describe what you experienced in writing.

Parent Note: You can talk your child through the creation of their happy place by asking them what they hear in this imaginary place, what they see, and so on.

What I heard:

_____

_____

_____

_____

What I saw:

_____

_____

_____

_____

What I felt:

_____

_____

_____

_____

What I tasted:

_____

_____

_____

_____

What I smelled:

_____

_____

_____

_____

Activity 3.29: Mindfulness Child Activity

Body Scan

Best for: All ages

Materials: None needed

Instructions for children: When you feel anxious, one way to make yourself feel better is to release the tension in your body. That's what the body scan helps you do. Lie down or sit comfortably in a chair. Close your eyes and take a minute to focus on your breath. Slowly breathe in through your nose and then out through your mouth. Starting at your toes, bring awareness into this part of your body for a few seconds. Focus on how your toes feel. Then begin to move up your body, stopping to take notice of feelings or sensations in each zone of your body (ankles, calves, thighs, hips, lower back, upper back, shoulders, neck, face, head). As you are focusing on each part of your body, take some deep breaths to encourage relaxation in that area. Then move on to the next body part and do the same.

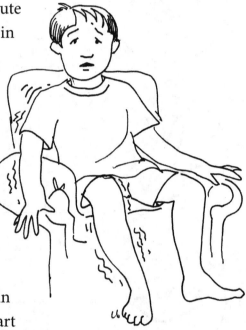

The best thing about a body scan is that it can be done anywhere. You do not need to lie or sit down to do it. You do not even have to close your eyes. You do not have to take big, obvious deep breaths. Wherever you are, when you begin to feel anxious, try to take a few minutes to take note of your body. If you feel tension in any area of your body, take a few deep breaths and release that tension, allowing it to melt away.

Activity 3.30: Mindfulness Child Activity*
Progressive Muscle Relaxation

Best for: All ages

Materials: None needed

Instructions for children: Progressive muscle relaxation is similar to body scanning (see Activity 3.29, Body Scan, p. 108). Progressive muscle relaxation is another way to relieve the tension that your body is holding. It can be especially helpful if you experience anxiety in your body, such as clenching your teeth or tensing your shoulders.

Begin by sitting comfortably in a chair and taking a few deep breaths. Then from the top of your head to the tips of your toes, tense and release different parts of your body. Start first with your jaw. Squeeze the muscles in your jaw as tight as you can for about five seconds and then release. Notice how much softer and calmer that part of your body feels. Next move on to your neck and shoulders. Bring your shoulders up to your ears and

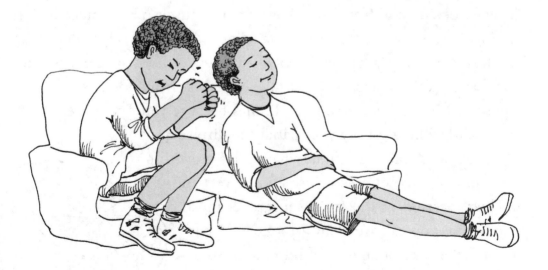

*Great for kids who experience physical tension such as increased heart rate, rapid breathing, and body tension

squeeze them, trying to touch the tops of your shoulders to your ears. Then release them and notice how relaxed your shoulders feel. Continue down through your body until you have tensed and released each part of your entire body. Take a few moments at the end to notice how your body feels once you have done this exercise.

This exercise can be done almost anywhere. You can tighten and release parts of your body in a way that is inconspicuous and others won't be able to tell what you are doing. This can be especially helpful if you experience physical symptoms of anxiety or if you are trying to disrupt obsessive thoughts.

Activity 3.31: Mindfulness Child Activity

Fresh Juice

Best for: Toddlers and preschoolers

Materials: Squeezable fruit such as a lemon, lime, or orange or a squeezable toy citrus fruit

Instructions for children: Fresh Juice is a fun muscle relaxation game (see Activity 3.30, Progressive Muscle Relaxation, p. 109) that can be done with real fruit or a squishy toy version of a fruit. If you choose a real fruit, pick one that typically squeezes to get juice. The best fruits for this are citrus fruits such as oranges, lemons, and limes because you can squeeze them really hard without getting your hands too dirty!

If you use a real fruit, cut it in half (ask a grown-up for help if you're not able to use a knife yet) and, holding the rind of the fruit, squeeze as much juice out as you can. You can get a bowl or cup to catch the juice or squeeze it into the trash or sink. If you are using a toy fruit, pretend you are squeezing out as much juice as possible. The

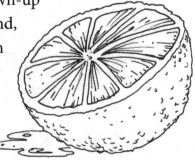

harder you squeeze your fruit, the more juice comes out. Sometimes even when you think that you've squeezed all the juice out, you can let the fruit rest, then squeeze again and it may produce more juice. Warning: If you use real fruit, you will get sticky! Have fun, but be careful not to rub your eyes!

You can also use pretend fruit for this exercise, but we recommend doing it a little differently if you do. Pretend you are holding a ripe orange in your hands. Squeeze the fruit as hard as you can. Pretend to make juice. Once your hands are tired out, squeeze the pretend fruit with your toes, between the knees, between your elbows, and more. Get creative!

Activity 3.32: Mindfulness Child Activity

Squeezy Sponge

Best for: Toddlers and preschoolers

Materials: Sponges, water, measuring cup (optional)

Instructions for children: Squeezy Sponge is another muscle relaxation game (see Activities 3.30, Progressive Muscle Relaxation, and 3.31, Fresh Juice, pp. 110 and 111). It can be messy, so make sure to get a grown-up to help you.

Get a clean sponge and a bucket of water. Put the sponge in the water and observe how it soaks it up. Remove the sponge and squeeze it out. Notice how the harder you squeeze, the more water comes out. Try out different ways of squeezing the sponge. Twisting the sponge or bunching it up are examples, but if you have other ideas, try them too! If you have

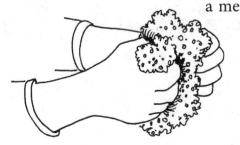

a measuring cup, squeeze the water into it and compare how much water you can get out with different types of squeezing. If your grown-up gives you permission, see what happens when you step on the sponge or squeeze it between your knees.

Activity 3.33: Mindfulness Child Activity

Calm Down Jar

Best for: Preschoolers, grade-school kids, and tweens

Materials: Jar, water, glitter glue

Instructions for children: This exercise combines a fun art project with a mindfulness exercise. Get a jar—preferably a nonbreakable one—and fill it almost to the top with water. Leave enough space to add two to three heaping spoonfuls of glitter glue. Shut or glue the lid on very tightly, making sure that no water or glitter glue can escape. *This step is very important or the exercise will be a total mess!*

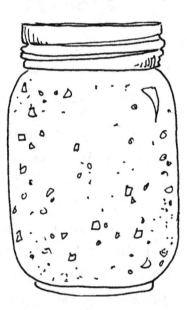

This jar is your calm down jar. When you are feeling stressed, get your calm down jar and sit in a comfortable, calm place. Shake the jar and watch the glitter fall to the bottom of the jar as you take deep calming breaths. Repeat as many times as necessary. (If you do not want to make your own calm down jar, you can also buy a snow globe. We recommend a large snow globe without a lot of distracting figures or words in it. You want the focus to be on the flakes as they fall to the bottom.)

Self-Regulation Interventions and Exercises

Remember: You do not need to try out all of these interventions and exercises.

The goal is to find a few that work well for your child.

Activity 3.34: Self-Regulation Child Activity

Give a Hug, Get a Hug

Best for: All ages

Materials: None needed

Instructions for children: Touch from a trusted person can be a very powerful calming tool. A strong hug can calm you down and reduce the physical symptoms of anxiety such as increased heart rate, rapid breathing, and body tension. When you feel anxious, ask for a strong hug from someone 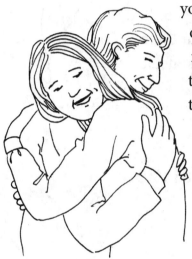 you know and trust. This can be a teacher, a friend, or a family member. If you are not comfortable receiving a hug in that moment or no one you trust is around, find a stuffed animal or pillow that you can squeeze. Or feel free to give yourself a hug. You can do this by wrapping your arms around your body and trying to touch your hands behind your back. This is very hard, if not impossible, for most people to do, but it will encourage you to really squeeze your body and help keep you calm in the moment.

Activity 3.35: Self-Regulation Child Activity

Get Twisty

Best for: All ages

Materials: None needed

Instructions for children: This exercise helps you loosen your body when it feels tense and tight. Raise your arms out in front of you at shoulder height. Cross your left elbow over your right elbow and then try to put your right wrist over your left wrist and grasp your fingers together. You will likely have to bend your arms to do this. If you can't grasp your hands together, that is fine. Now cross your legs and twist them around themselves. This is known as Eagle Pose in yoga. If this pose does not feel good to you, feel free to twist your body in another way. You don't need to strain in this exercise. You should not feel any pain or discomfort. Twist or contort your body as much as you are able, but do not hurt yourself! Try to hold this twisted position for one minute. When our bodies are twisted we tend to hold our breath, so remember to breathe! Keep breathing deeply during this time. After a minute passes, unwind your body and continue breathing deeply, noticing that your body is looser and more in control. This can be done seated or standing. (It depends on your balance skills!)

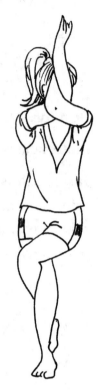

Activity 3.36: Self-Regulation Child Activity

Cold Drink of Water

Samantha's Top Pick

Best for: All ages

Materials: Cold water

Instructions for children: This exercise is exactly what it sounds like. When you find yourself experiencing the physical signs of anxiety such as increased heart rate, rapid breathing, sweating, or body tension, go and get a cold drink of water. Drinking the water will help regulate your breathing and relax your body. It is hard to drink when your breathing is shallow! The cold temperature can shock your system or distract you. This can help you recognize how tense you are. After a few shallow sips, allow yourself to take a long, deep drink. When you are done, let out a long breath and say

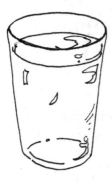

"ahhhh"—just like in a soft drink commercial! This will also slow your breathing down. Best of all, this can be done almost anywhere. If this is an effective strategy for you, it can be a good idea to bring a cold bottle of water with you to places where you expect you'll experience anxiety.

Activity 3.37: Self-Regulation Child Activity

Exercise!

Best for: All ages

Materials: None needed

Instructions for children: Research has proven time and again that physical exercise can decrease feelings of anxiety and improve overall mood by releasing endorphins. Endorphins are natural chemicals our bodies produce that make us happy! Some studies have shown exercise to be more effective than medication in reducing stress!

In this intervention, we're simply encouraging you to get moving! Use the strength and power you feel while exercising as a reminder that you are powerful and in control of your own body and mind. Here are a few ideas of what to do to start moving your body and reducing your anxiety:

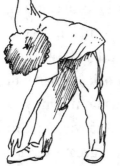
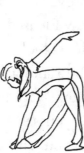

Run	Jump	Skip
Hop	Swim	Scoot
Skate	Yoga	Box
Walk	Bounce	Dance
Push-ups	Climb	Jump rope
Bike	Paddle	Swing
Jumping jacks		

Activity 3.38: Self-Regulation Child Activity

Stress Balls!

Best for: All ages

Materials: Squeeze ball or balloon and a selection of miscellaneous objects

Instructions for children: Make or buy a stress ball and carry it with you wherever you go. When you begin to feel your anxiety rising, reach for your stress ball and start squeezing. As you squeeze, feel the tension in your arm build and then notice your muscles relax as you release. If you'd like, switch hands every once in a while.

If you choose to make your own squeeze ball, a balloon is a good "skin." Here are some options for materials to fill your balloon:

Sand	Slime	Flour	Rice
Cornstarch	Beans	Baking soda	Hair conditioner

Activity 3.39: Self-Regulation Child Activity

Fidgeting

Best for: All ages

Materials: Fidget spinner, a smooth rock, a small ball of clay, pipe cleaners, rubber bands, or a few coins

Instructions for children: Fidgeting has been proven to be a helpful calming tool. Fidgeting can also help some people to stay focused. In this intervention, we suggest making, finding, or buying a "fidget tool." A fidget tool could be a store-bought fidget spinner, but it can also be a smooth rock, a small ball of clay, pipe cleaners, rubber bands, or a few coins. Have this item with you or nearby (whenever it is allowed) and remind yourself that if you start to feel overwhelmed, you have a calming tool with you. This is a great exercise

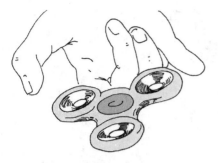

to combine with another intervention—for example, when you touch your fidget it can become a cue to take a few deep breaths (see Activity 3.22, Deep Breathing Basics, p. 99) or do a body scan (see Activity 3.29, Body Scan, p. 108).

Parent Note: Some schools do not allow children to have some of these items. Please check your school's policies and choose an item that your school allows, or obtain special permission if needed.

Activity 3.40: Self-Regulation Child Activity

Just Listen (or Sing Too)

*Melissa's Top Pick

Best for: All ages

Materials: Speaker or phone to play music, paper, and pen (optional)

Instructions for children: Research shows that music engages many different parts of the brain and can help to lower cortisol levels and reduce anxiety.[1] (Cortisol is a chemical your body produces when it is stressed out.) Therefore, music can be a very effective relaxation aid. In this intervention, we recommend that you listen to some favorite tunes. Pick one or a few songs that help you feel calm or help you release tension. Listen to this music when you feel your anxiety increasing.

Singing is also helpful as a relaxation tool because it helps to regulate breathing and requires attention from different areas of the brain. This means that when you are singing, you don't have time to worry about other things! As a bonus exercise, write down the lyrics to your favorite songs and keep them somewhere you can easily access them (like in a small journal

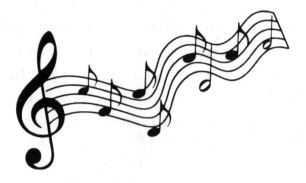

or on an index card). Pick a few favorite lines and use them as mantras to memorize. (A mantra is a sound, statement, or slogan that you can recite to help focus your thoughts and feelings.)

Activity 3.41: Self-Regulation Child Activity

Take-a-Break Bowl

Best for: All ages

Materials: Bowl, pen or pencil, paper

Instructions for children: This exercise challenges you to think about all the different things that make you feel calm. Sometimes when we're upset it is hard to remember the things that help to relax you. This exercise helps you access those ideas when you need them the most.

On separate pieces of paper, write down or draw each thing that helps calm you when you are anxious or upset. You can even include some of the worksheets in this chapter! It is most helpful if the calming things you choose are easily accessible and doable almost anywhere. For example, cuddling with a stuffed animal is easier to access than going to a favorite amusement park, though you could write down something like "pretending I'm at the amusement park" like you did in the visualization intervention (see Activity 3.27, Visualization, p. 105). Once you have all your ideas written or drawn on paper, place the sheets of paper in a bowl. Keep the bowl in a safe and reachable place. When you are upset, you can

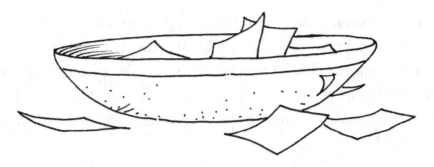

come and pick out a piece of paper (no peeking) and try the activity that's on it. If you want, you can ask a grown-up to remind you to visit the bowl when you need to.

Activity 3.42: Self-Regulation Child Activity

Just Talk . . .

Best for: All ages

Materials: Someone/something you trust

Instructions for children: Talking helps! It may seem obvious, but we can all use a reminder of this simple fact. Sometimes things seem way worse in our minds than they do in reality. Talking through a fear, worry, or negative experience can help you release your feelings of worry instead of holding on to them.

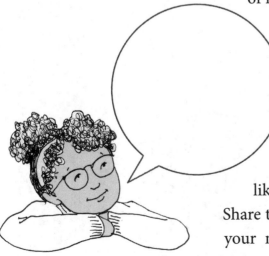

Start by finding a good listener. This can be an actual person, but it can also be a pet, a stuffed animal, or a plant or a tree. (Did you know that talking to plants can help them grow!)[2] You can also talk to a loved one who has died, like a grandmother you were close to. Share the thoughts and worries that are on your mind. If you're comfortable, move into problem-solving mode by asking the person for advice or telling them what you are going to do to make a problem better. Remember, just because someone offers advice doesn't mean you have to take it. Sometimes hearing an idea that doesn't sit well with you is just as helpful as hearing one that does. You don't necessarily have to take any action at all. Sometimes talking is all you need.

Activity 3.43: Self-Regulation Child Activity
Blow!

Best for: All ages (especially young children)

Materials: Be creative

Instructions for children: Breathing is one of the best ways to regulate your body but, for many of us, deep breathing exercises are not easy to do. Or sometimes they just don't seem to help. In this exercise, the idea is to blow your breath out for as long as you can. You can practice this many ways. You can blow bubbles, pinwheels, spinning fans, candles, dandelion seeds—anything that reacts to your efforts! Test out different bubble wands. Use relighting candles. Have fun! Be creative with it! Time yourself (or have a grown-up time you) to see how long you can exhale.

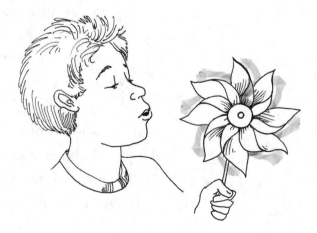

Activity 3.44: Self-Regulation Child Activity

Stuffed Animal Snuggle

Best for: Toddlers and preschoolers

Materials: A favorite stuffed animal

Instructions for children: Pick a stuffed animal that you love. It can be one that you already have or a brand new one. Put the stuffed animal in a special place in your room. When you are feeling overwhelmed or frustrated, give the stuffed animal a big squeeze. You can also tell your stuffed animal what you are thinking and feeling. Let the animal hear about what has been happening and what you are worried about. But you don't have to talk to your stuffed animal if you don't want to. You can just sit there, giving your stuffed animal a hug and allowing it to comfort you. This can also be done with a blankie or other comfort object. The stuffed animal is there to help you keep calm (or calm down if you've already become upset) and provide support.

Creativity Interventions and Exercises

Remember: You do not need to try out all of these interventions and exercises.

The goal is to find a few that work well for your child.

Activity 3.45: Creativity Child Activity

Draw Your Anxiety

Best for: All ages

Materials: Drawing materials

Instructions for children: This exercise helps to explore what anxiety means for you. Draw a picture of your anxiety. Use the whole space to express what it looks like to you. Perhaps it's a figure, like a cloud or a monster. Or it may just be a group of lines and scribbles. There's no right or wrong! And keep in mind that working with your hands is a good stress reliever. This exercise helps you to release tension while you are gaining more understanding of your anxiety.

Activity 3.46: Creativity Child Activity

Anxiety in Your Body

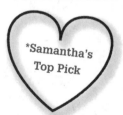

*Samantha's Top Pick

Best for: All ages

Materials: Butcher/utility paper, drawing materials

Instructions for children: Get a really large piece of paper (bigger and wider than you are) and lie down on it. Ask someone to draw an outline of your body on the paper. Now look at the picture of your body and consider where and how you experience anxiety in your body. Grab your drawing materials and label or draw where you feel anxiety. Use a color or image that represents what your anxiety feels like. What might it look like in your body? How would you describe these feelings to someone (parent, sibling, friend)? Remember, exploring your personal experience of anxiety helps you learn how to best manage it.

Activity 3.47: Creativity Child Activity

Child-Driven Time

Melissa's Top Pick

Best for: All ages

Materials: Perhaps some toys

Instructions for parents: Parents, this one is for you! Child-driven time or "special time" is a method that, when done earnestly, almost always brings noticeable results. The idea here is that you are creating meaningful positive connection with your child. You may spend quite a bit of time with your child as it is, but how often are you completely focused on them with the intention of connecting? Set aside a ten- to fifteen-minute window that is centered around your child. Daily would be great, but we know that's not always possible so we suggest aiming for at least two times per week. Make sure you designate the day and time to keep it consistent and sacred.

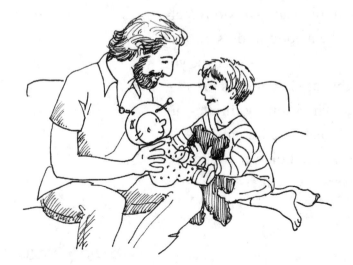

During this time, all attention is on your child. (Yes, put down that phone and turn the ringer and notifications off!) Set a timer and engage in whatever play your child chooses during the time. Your child is completely in charge of how you two entertain yourselves and gets to direct everything (within basic safety constraints, of course). They decide what you are playing, who plays what role, what you say, and so on, and you just play along.

> **Parent Note:** Child-driven time is a one-on-one experience. If you have more than one child, special time should be devoted to each one individually. Also, for older children/teens, the time together may be less play focused but it should still be child-led one-on-one time.

Activity 3.48: Creativity Child Activity

Samantha's Top Pick

Exploring Your Anxiety

Best for: Grade-school kids, tweens, and teens

Materials: Drawing materials

Instructions for children: One of the first steps in managing anxious feelings is having a good understanding of those feelings. In this exercise you explore what anxiety means for you.

This activity is pretty simple—just answer the following imaginative questions. Draw a picture to illustrate your answers if you like.

What color is my anxiety?

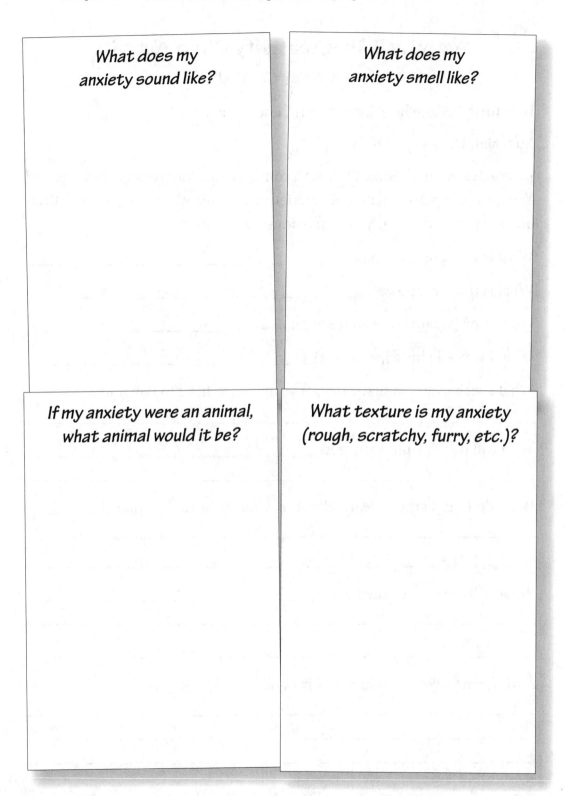

*What does my
anxiety sound like?*

*What does my
anxiety smell like?*

*If my anxiety were an animal,
what animal would it be?*

*What texture is my anxiety
(rough, scratchy, furry, etc.)?*

Activity 3.49: Creativity Child Activity

Anxiety Comics!

Best for: Grade-school kids, tweens, and teens

Material: Drawing materials

Instructions for children: Create a comic of you conquering your anxiety! You are the superhero and your anxiety is the villain. Answer the questions on this page and on the next page draw your comic!

What is my superhero name?_____

What is my superpower? _____

What is my villain's (my anxiety's) name? _____

What is my villain's superpower? _____

What specific anxiety/issue does my superhero have to conquer?

_____

Who will help me on my quest? _____

_____

What do I (and others) learn about my villain during my quest? _____

_____

_____

What will the next challenge be? _____

_____

_____

Additional things to include in my comic:

_____

_____

_____

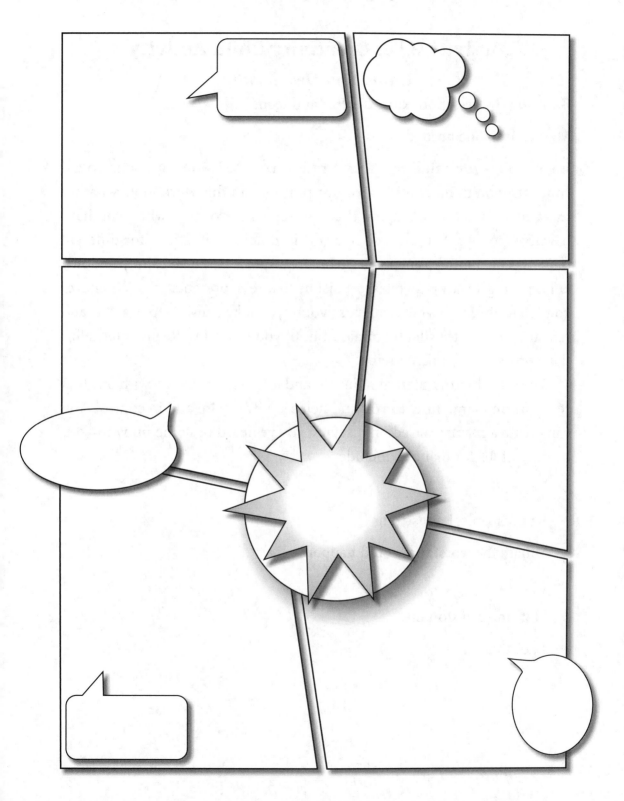

Activity 3.50: Creativity Child Activity

Create Your Own Mantra

Best for: Grade-school kids, tweens, and teens

Materials: None needed

Instructions for children: A mantra is a repeated word or sound to aid concentration in meditation. For our purposes in this workbook, what we call a mantra is a short saying that you repeat to yourself when you have negative feelings. You can use mantras in different situations for different purposes, including to pep you up before a sports game, to calm you down before a big test, or to release tension before a presentation. Whenever you are feeling overwhelmed, close your eyes, take a few deep breaths, and repeat your mantra silently or aloud until you feel calm. Really internalize the word(s) that you are saying.

There are lots of different mantras, and it's best to come up with one that really means something to you and helps you feel calm and in control. You can create a mantra based on a saying you've heard or come up with your own. Options for mantras include:

❖ I can do it.

❖ I am capable. I am strong.

❖ What's the worst that could happen?

❖ I'm ready.

❖ Nothing can stop me.

❖ I got this.

When you have determined what your mantra should be, write it down in a place (or places) where you will see it every day. Here are some options for where to put your mantra:

❖ Create a picture with your mantra, frame it, and hang it on your bedroom wall.

❖ Write your mantra on the inside cover of your notebook or binder.

❖ Write your mantra on the inside of the tongue of your favorite sneakers. (You'll see it each time you lace up!)

❖ Pin it up above the area where you wash your face and hands, do your hair, brush your teeth, put on makeup, etc.

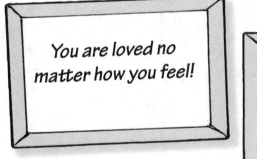

4

Maintenance: Maintaining and Gaining

Chapter Introduction

You have arrived at the maintenance chapter! Chapter 2, "Parent Prep," and chapter 3, "Interventions," really focus on skills you and your child can use to cope with anxiety. This chapter combines individual gains with the gains of the larger family unit. No child is an island, and the actions of each family member influence everyone else in the family. Our hope is that in working with this book, all family members become more aware of their own feelings, thoughts, and behaviors and how they affect others. Increased awareness of your feelings is the first step to controlling them. This applies to every family member. By putting interventions in place that target the whole family, as opposed to just one person, you are sending the message that everyone can benefit from this work (which is true) and that the child who is struggling does not have to do it all on their own (also true).

You may be thinking there are so many interventions in chapter 3 and you've tried a bunch of them with success. Why do you need to do more? That's a good question! The interventions in this chapter are part of what we call your maintenance plan. Research shows that the gains kids make when working on their emotional struggles are more successful when parents are involved in the process.[1] However, parents can't make everything better all on their own. It is also vital that parents empower children to make decisions regarding their emotional lives. Essentially, parents have an important, but complicated, role to play in maintaining their children's gains. You want to provide support, but not take over. The first step to achieving the right balance between support and empowerment is understanding the concept of maintenance.

Defining Maintenance

We define successful maintenance as the process that occurs when a person can recognize anxiety triggers and symptoms, utilize coping skills, and adapt as necessary—*most of the time.* That "most of the time" part is really important. Life happens, and there are times when things just feel like too much. We know there will be times when it feels impossible to keep your stuff together! So remember that we are not aiming for perfection. We repeat: *we are not aiming for perfection.* Now that we've made that clear, let's break down what maintenance entails.

Recognize Triggers and Symptoms

You want your child to know when they are experiencing anxiety. The goal is for them to know what happens in their bodies when their anxiety is out of control. Are they able to identify when they feel anxious and why? Is there something that consistently triggers feelings of anxiety for them? What do they feel like when that happens?

There will always be times when something new pops up that causes anxiety and children are unable to anticipate their reactions. There are a number of things that could come up and change how your child's anxiety manifests. Moreover, your child may simply have an off day that leads to them forgetting their triggers and symptoms. That's okay! Everyone has an off day once in a while. But if your child has a basic understanding of their anxiety and recognizes their symptoms and triggers *most of the time*, they are moving toward the maintenance phase.

Utilize Coping Skills

In addition to being able to recognize their symptoms of anxiety, you also want your child to be able to do something about them. A child may know what is happening but then become paralyzed and unable to act to mitigate those symptoms. Or they may attempt to use coping skills that are not working for them. Some kids may be taught deep breathing or meditation-type skills at school or during other activities. This is great if the tools work for your child. But if they don't work, or only work temporarily, your child needs other options that will truly do the job. In other words, when your child is able to keep calm or calm down enough that their anxiety does not negatively impact their day, then they are experiencing successful signs of maintenance.

Kids aren't *always* going to be able to use the coping skills they have. Sometimes a given situation is too overwhelming, consuming, or emotional and all logical thought goes out the window. At other times, your child may be collected enough to try a number of coping skills but none of the skills work. This can happen even if those same coping skills worked in the past. Help your child not to see this as failure, nor as a sign that these coping skills will no longer work at all. Although this might be the case, it may also be that this coping skill just didn't work this time or in this situation. If your child's coping skills are working most of the time, in the majority of settings, or just in the most important settings (at school, in front of friends, in a high-stakes situation), then your child is likely moving successfully into the maintenance phase.

Adapt as Necessary

Now your child can (mostly) recognize their symptoms and (mostly) utilize their coping skills to calm themselves down. The third element of maintenance is successfully adjusting and adapting to new situations. But what happens when new symptoms pop up or a coping skill stops working (not just once but several times in a row)? Does your child try (in vain) to keep using the same coping skill even though it is clearly not working? Does your child ignore the fact that they are experiencing new symptoms? Or is your child able to recognize that something new has popped up and they need to problem-solve? If you're not sure how to respond to these questions, that's okay! But if you think you can answer yes to at least one of them, this is a sign that your child is in maintenance. Remember, what you are looking for is your child to be able to adjust and adapt to new situations. You want them to be able to recognize when something isn't working and to make a shift.

As with the other elements of maintenance, you can't expect that a child is always going to recognize that they need something more or different in a given situation. Doing that is a challenge even for adults, and that's just not how the developing brain works. It will likely take your child a little longer than it would an adult to realize this new situation may be taking a negative emotional toll. (Although some children are actually *better* at this than adults!) Your child may need you to gently point out that some new or changed circumstances or situation may be impacting how they feel. If your child is able to listen to you and adapt accordingly or make changes on their own most of the time, they are *definitely* moving toward maintenance.

Involving Others—Revisited

As authors, we debated whether to include this section because the decision to involve other people and which people to involve in the maintenance phase is really up to you. On the one hand, just like in the interventions phase (as we discussed in chapter 2), it may be helpful for significant adults in your child's life to be involved in the maintenance phase. Their involvement helps a child to feel supported and to practice the coping skills at times when you (the parent) are not around. However, the maintenance phase is a little different from the intervention phase. Although having important adults continue to be involved may lead to more success, at some point you may want to taper off reliance on others. Eventually your child will be in settings and situations where not everyone will be accommodating toward them. This may occur in high school, college, grad school, or the workplace. It may be good for your child to experience what life will be like when everyone around them is not aware of and part of a plan to support them. At a certain point, your child will have to manage their own anxiety primarily on their own.

So the answer about whether to involve other people in the maintenance phase is the always infuriating: *it depends*. Though we can't give you a concrete answer about whom to involve, we can provide you with some questions to ask yourself that may make your decision a little easier.

1. *How old is your child?* If your child is a teenager, you may want to involve only the people that absolutely need to know. This is not because their anxiety is a secret but because your child will be out on their own before you know it and will need to be managing as much as possible on their own.

2. *How long has your child been experiencing anxiety? How severe is their anxiety?* If anxiety is something they have always dealt with and is relatively low level, then others may not need to be involved. However, if your child's anxiety is something that has come on fast and furiously or is very acute, you may want some extra support to help keep the intensity of flare-ups to a minimum.

3. *Has your child been using coping skills consistently and regularly?* If your child is doing relatively well most of the time (see p. 132), then others may not need to be involved in maintenance.

4. *Where does your child experience anxiety?* Does your child have the majority of symptoms at home, at school, at sports practice, while socializing with friends? If they manage their anxiety well at school

and at basketball practice and experience anxiety flare-ups primarily at home, there is no need to involve teachers and coaches.

5. *Does your child embarrass easily or have they expressed that they do not want others to know?* This is *so important*. Involving others is only helpful if the child doesn't fight against it. If you find that your child's embarrassment is stronger than their anxiety, you may not want to involve others. Doing so may increase their feelings of shame and may make the anxiety worse.

6. *Have you asked your child if they want to involve others?* This question seems obvious, but we often overlook this. What does your child think? It is their life, after all. This may end up being the only question that really matters.

Developing a Maintenance Plan

It's exciting if you are feeling you've finally landed in the maintenance phase. Things are going pretty well. Your child has some coping skills and is using those skills on a regular basis. There have been some flare-ups, but nothing like you've previously seen. After looking at the definition of maintenance on page 132 and asking yourself the necessary questions to see if others need to be involved on page 53, you are ready to develop your own maintenance plan! Congratulations—you and your child have really earned this!

So what is a maintenance plan? In this book it is more than just a thought exercise; it is a document that you fill out to help keep track of how things are going. It is a place to list the interventions that are working and those you tried that really didn't do the job. It is also a place to document how family members—and any others you may choose—will continue to be involved and provide support.

Work with your child to complete the maintenance plan on the following pages. The plan will help you both keep track of your child's progress. We also highly recommend using this form to celebrate successes.

Celebrations can be almost anything, but don't underestimate the power of praise. Let your kid know when they are doing a good job and that you are proud of them. Even if they are doing just what you'd expect, it's still important to praise their efforts. Do this often. Praise can be a huge motivator.

However you choose to celebrate your child, make sure it is motivating to *them* and appropriate for their age. For example, it can be great to praise your five-year-old in front of their teacher. The same thing might make your fifteen-year-old die of embarrassment, but they may appreciate a quick text with a silly emoji. And every once in a while, surprising a kid of any age with a trip to their favorite ice cream shop can make them feel special. Be creative with how you utilize your maintenance plan and you'll continue to see your child's successes grow and multiply.

This section has six additional maintenance phase activities that reinforce the success and support your child has had thus far. We call these family activities, but they can apply to other groups—friends, extended family members, a sports team, and so on. They can also be done independently if that works best for your child.

Family Interventions and Exercises

Activity 4.1: Maintenance Family Activity
Maintenance Plan

This exercise is a living document of the plan for how to maintain the gains that you and your child (and spouse . . . and other child . . . and grandmother . . . and . . .) have made. You have worked hard—you don't want to forget it all! Fill in the blanks on the next three pages to document what has gone well and what hasn't, as well as ways to provide support and areas where you want to continue to grow. Writing it all down makes it easier to remember what you've done and to celebrate your accomplishments!

These are the interventions that work for us:

Write the names of the activities and/or page numbers from the previous chapter. If you have other go-to interventions, feel free to list those here too.

1. _____

_____

2. _____

_____

3. _____

_____

4. _____

These are the interventions that have not worked for us:

Write the names of the activities and/or page numbers from the previous chapter.

1. _____

_____

2. _____

_____

3. _____

_____

4. _____

These are examples of support provided by the family:

How have family members helped your child? Has your daughter gently nudged her brother when she notices he may benefit from some deep breathing? Have parents allowed their teen to download helpful apps? Did Dad trace his daughter for Activity 3.46, Anxiety in Your Body (p. 122)? These seemingly small supports likely helped in a big way and should be recognized.

_____

_____

_____

_____

_____

These are examples of support provided by others:

Were there friends who checked in on your child? Or a coach who allowed your child to have a fidget spinner even though it is usually not allowed? What about teachers who helped your child manage their anxiety symptoms? Write these down as well.

_____

_____

_____

_____

_____

How long has our child used their successful coping skills consistently?

Skill _____ weeks/months _____

Skill _____ weeks/months _____

Skill _____ weeks/months _____

Skill _____ weeks/months _____

These are the areas that still need work:

Are there places that are still a struggle? Do many of the interventions work but you feel they need tweaking?

_____

_____

_____

_____

_____

_____

These are additional interventions/coping skills we may want to try:

_____

_____

_____

_____

_____

_____

These are our successes!

What "wins" have you felt or seen since you began to work through the anxiety? List them all out—big and small.

_____

_____

_____

_____

_____

_____

Activity 4.2: Maintenance Family Activity
Relaxation Haven

Instructions: Have each family member find a place in the house that can become a space just for them. This can be an entire room if space permits or a small, cozy corner if that is more practical. This space is each individual's "relaxation haven." It is a space where only that person can go, and the only thing they will do in that space is relax. Once each space is identified and communicated to the rest of the family, each person can fill their own space with things that are relaxing to them. Feel free to decorate your space with colors and items that you love. Get creative! Reminders and instructions for additional relaxing activities can be included in your space as well. This isn't a place to play video games, work on school projects, hang out with friends, or do your taxes. If you have something in the space that you want others to use—such as a beanbag chair—it can be moved to another part of the room when you are not in your haven. By keeping each space sacred, each person will start to calm down more quickly when they seek refuge in their space.

Here are some suggestions for things to put in a relaxation haven:

❖ Books

❖ Lamps with dim lightbulbs

❖ A beanbag chair

❖ Fluffy pillows

❖ Blankets

❖ A stuffed animal (see Activity 3.44, Stuffed Animal Snuggle, p. 121)

❖ Cards with breathing exercises on them (see Activity 3.22, Deep Breathing Basics, p. 99)

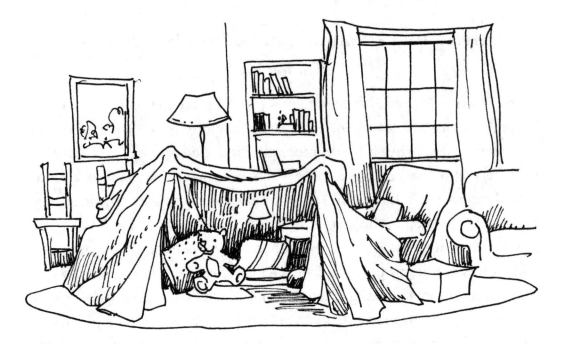

❖ Headphones and your favorite visualization audio (see Activity 3.27, Visualization, p. 105)

❖ A sign with your favorite mantra (see Activity 3.50, Create Your Own Mantra, p. 128)

❖ An electronic water fountain

❖ Slippers or cozy socks

Activity 4.3: Maintenance Family Activity

Coping Skills Toolbox

Instructions: By this time, the person in the family who is experiencing anxiety—and hopefully others in the family as well—has tried many different coping skills. Some have worked well and others have not. Not everything works for everyone. It is a good idea to keep track of the coping skills that were successful so that it is easier to remember to use them—even when people are upset. Have each person in the family make their own

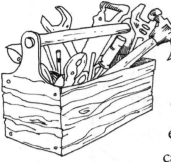

coping skills toolbox and/or you can have a family coping skills toolbox that anyone can use.

To make a coping skills toolbox, take a large jar or box and decorate it. Label it "Coping Skills Toolbox." Inside, place things that are good reminders of your successful and useful coping skills. This can include pictures of calming places, links to sites for meditation and visualization, cards with instructions, a stress ball, a journal (best for an individual coping skills toolbox), and so forth. Once you decorate and fill the toolbox(es), store in a private but easily accessible place. If each person has their own toolbox, have a time every week for everyone to pull out their boxes and dig in! During that weekly session, each person can look at the items already in their box as reminders and perhaps add more coping skill reminders. Individuals can also use their boxes anytime on an as-needed basis. If you have a family toolbox, take it out once a week to do the same thing, or just use it whenever someone needs it.

Activity 4.4: Maintenance Family Activity

Family Mantra

Instructions: This activity is similar to Activity 3.50, Create Your Own Mantra (p. 128), except this time the entire family creates a family mantra. Recall that in this workbook, what we call a mantra is a short saying that you can repeat to yourself when you have negative feelings. This mantra is representative of who you all are as a family and the values that you hold. It also helps remind individual family members who are struggling with anxiety (or anything else) that the family is there to support them.

Your family mantra can be a saying that someone already uses or something that everyone comes up with together. Post your family mantra somewhere in the house where everyone in the family can see it. This can be discreet or as bold and open as you choose. Make the commitment as a family

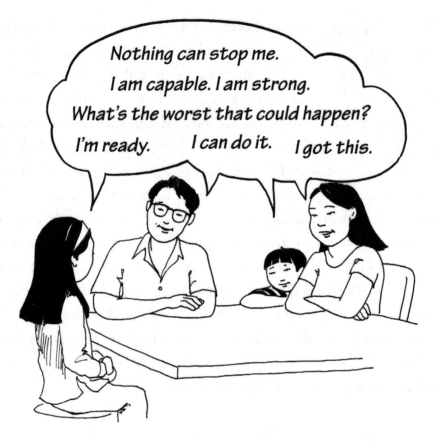

to say this phrase often, especially during times when you know a member of the family needs support. Recognize that this won't necessarily change anyone's mood completely, but it can help family members feel supported or trigger them to use the coping skills they've developed (see Activity 4.3, Coping Skills Toolbox, pp. 142–143).

Creating a family mantra is a good way to open up a conversation about how we all struggle with something. Whether we are experiencing anxiety, depression, stress, or exhaustion, we all need a boost every once in a while. As you work to figure out your family mantra, have everyone in the family express what they identify as their most acute struggle and express when they may need to hear that family mantra. Allow everyone to talk about how the mantra makes them feel and what it does for them.

Activity 4.5: Maintenance Family Activity

Family Meeting

Instructions: Assigning a regular time when the family gets together to talk about concerns can be a really positive practice. It allows each member of the family to celebrate things that are going well ("I used my stress ball during my exam and was able to complete the whole test without panicking!") as well as areas where individuals need support ("I'm struggling to remember to take deep breaths when I feel my heart racing before a big game"). A family meeting signals that all problems can be tackled together, and even if you can't solve them, there may be things that can be done to make them better. Parents sharing some of their struggles and frustrations (appropriately, of course) is a great way to model that everyone has things that are hard for them and even as adults we have to work through these things.

The family meeting can be very structured or relatively casual, depending on your family's needs. We recommend starting with a more structured

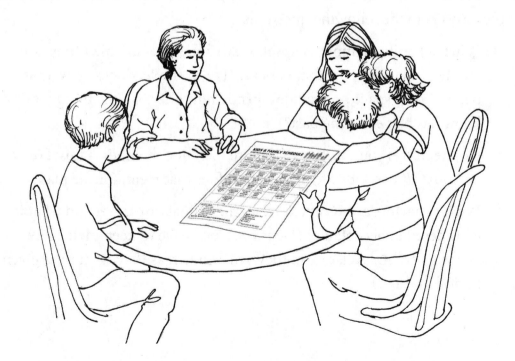

format and then moving to a more relaxed style (it's harder to transition from less structure to more). Below is a sample agenda for a family meeting:

Have everyone share a success from the past week.

❖ Have each person share one thing that they need to problem-solve or would like support around.

❖ Spend five minutes on each person's concern and offering suggestions and support.

❖ End with saying something positive about the past week and the person on your right.

Activity 4.6: Maintenance Family Activity

Family Calm Down Rules

Instructions: Meet as a family (preferably within a family meeting; see Activity 4.5, Family Meeting, p. 145–146) and establish some family rules for handling anxiety. To do this, get a large sheet of paper and write down the answers to the following questions:

❖ When a family member is upset or anxious, what are the things the family does to support that person? (For example, do you give that person some space or provide a gentle reminder of something you know has helped in the past?)

❖ Do the things you do change if more than one member is upset or anxious? (If two kids are upset, what does that mean for the plan?)

❖ What behaviors are accepted when individuals are upset and what is considered unacceptable? (Does everyone have to keep their voice below a certain level, or can they yell as much as they want for a given period of time?)

Think about examples of times when a family member was struggling and discuss what others did to help. Feel free to use examples where things went terribly wrong! Thinking about what does and does not work will help prompt discussions about what to include in your rules if the family gets stumped. Make sure that everyone in the family contributes and feels as if their voices are heard. There may be disagreement about what is considered acceptable—that is okay. Feel free to use the interventions from chapter 3 as guides. For example, family members can encourage each other to reframe (Activity 3.14, Reframing, p. 84), engage in ACT behaviors (Activity 3.13, ACT [Acknowledge, Consider, Try], p. 82), and plan for the problem (Activity 3.18, Plan for the "Problem," p. 90) when faced with disagreements or stressful situations.

5

Resources

Chapter Introduction

You did it—you finished the book! Well, almost. All that's left now are lists of additional tools and resources. Did you make it through from start to finish, or are you just popping into chapter 5 to see what else is out there? Either way, we are glad you're here. We want you to take a moment and reflect on *why* you are here. If you *have* read the book and tried some interventions, you may have read references to a few helpful supplements and additional resources back here. If you've skipped ahead to this chapter, take a look around and see what jumps out. Please know that we believe everything listed in this chapter can be helpful, but unfortunately there are no easy outs. These resources are great, but they are not substitutes for doing the work in the activities and the detailed information we've provided in chapters 1 through 4.

We know this workbook has a lot of information and we've asked a lot of you. We've challenged you to reflect on yourself, introduced you to over fifty interventions for you and your family, and now we're listing a bunch of other ideas. We do not want to overwhelm you, but we do want you to have resources available if and when you need them.

We also offer the suggestions in table 5.1 for reviewing the resources.

Table 5.1 Anxiety Reduction Resource Dos and Don'ts

Do check out or put a few of the adult books on hold at your local library. Read through them one at a time slowly, and don't worry about memorizing all the information.	**Don't** read four of the children's books to your child in one sitting; they may start to feel shame about their anxiety or see it as a burden.
Do explore some of the relaxation apps and choose one so you or your child have access to them even when away from home.	**Don't** give up on an app or a game because it wasn't a hit the first time; try again in a few weeks or months.
Do give yourself a pat on the back. You are a rock star parent! Not only did you identify a concern but you bought and read this entire book to try and address your concerns. *And* you're considering even more resources.	**Don't** feel like you need to read and research every resource available about childhood anxiety all at once. You've read this book, and these other resources aren't going anywhere!

Books about Anxiety for All Ages

We are big advocates for reading other books in addition to our own! As amazing as we think this book is, we know we can't provide everything you may need. It can be helpful to read things from a variety of perspectives and/or to have your child read something themselves to really make all this helpful information stick. There are new books related to anxiety for adults and children coming out all the time, so this list is not comprehensive, but we've provided a few ideas here to get you started.

For Parents/Caregivers/Adults

❖ *Anxiety Relief for Kids: On-the-Spot Strategies to Help Your Child Overcome Worry, Panic, and Avoidance* by Bridget Flynn Walker

❖ *Freeing Your Child from Anxiety, Revised and Updated Edition: Practical Strategies to Overcome Fears, Worries, and Phobias and Be Prepared for Life—from Toddlers to Teens* by Tamar Chansky

❖ *Growing Up Brave: Expert Strategies for Helping Your Child Overcome Fear, Stress, and Anxiety* by Donna B. Pincus

❖ *Helping Your Anxious Child: A Step-by-Step Guide for Parents* by Ronald Rapee, Ann Wignall, Susan Spence, Vanessa Cobham, and Heidi Lyneham

❖ *The Whole Brain Child: 12 Revolutionary Strategies to Nurture Your Child's Developing Mind* by Daniel Siegel and Tina Payne Bryson

❖ *Why Smart Kids Worry: And What Parents Can Do to Help* by Allison Edwards

For Kids Age 8 and Under

❖ *A Terrible Thing Happened* by Margaret Holmes and Sasha Mudlaff

❖ *Be Kind* by Pat Zietlow Miller and Jen Hill

❖ *Big Brave Bold Sergio* by Debbie Wagenbach and Jamie Tablason

❖ *The Breaking News* by Sarah Lynne Reul

❖ *Breathe* by Iñes Castel-Branco

❖ *The Chocolate-Covered Cookie Tantrum* by Deborah Blumenthal and Harvey Stevenson

❖ *David and the Worry Beast: Helping Children Cope with Anxiety* by Anne Marie Guanci and Caroline Attia

❖ *Don't Think about Purple Elephants* by Susanne Merritt and Gwynneth Jones

❖ *I Walk With Vanessa: A Story about a Simple Act of Kindness* by Kerascoët

❖ *Is a Worry Worrying You?* by Ferida Wolff, Harriet May Savitz, and Marie Letourneau

❖ *Julián Is a Mermaid* by Jessica Love

❖ *Little Mouse's Big Book of Fears* by Emily Gravett

❖ *Mr. Worry: A Story about OCD* by Holly Niner and Greg Swearingen

❖ *My Somebody Special* by Sarah Weeks and Ashley Wolff

❖ *Silly Billy* by Anthony Browne

❖ *The Invisible String* by Patrice Karst and Joanne Lew-Vriethoff

❖ *The Kissing Hand* by Audrey Penn, Ruth Harper, and Nancy Leak

❖ *Storytime: The Otter Who Loved to Hold Hands* by Heidi and Daniel Howarth

❖ *The Worry Glasses: Overcoming Anxiety* by Donalisa Helsley and Kalpart

❖ *Wemberly Worried* by Kevin Henkes

❖ *When I Miss You* by Cornelia Maude Spelman and Kathy Parkinson

❖ *When My Worries Get Too Big!* by Kari Dunn Buron

❖ *When Sophie Gets Angry—Really, Really Angry . . .* by Molly Bang

For Kids Age 8–12

❖ *But What If?* by Sue Graves and Desideria Guicciardini

❖ *Hey Warrior* by Karen Young

❖ *Stress Can Really Get on Your Nerves* by Trevor Romain and Elizabeth Verdick

❖ *There's a Bully in My Brain* by Kristin O'Rourke

❖ *What to Do When You're Scared and Worried: A Guide for Kids* by James J. Crist

❖ *What to Do When You Worry Too Much: A Kid's Guide to Overcoming Anxiety* by Dawn Huebner

❖ *Wilma Jean—the Worry Machine* by Julia Cook and Anita DuFalla

For Kids Age 12 and Older

❖ *Anxiety Relief for Teens: Essential CBT Skills and Mindfulness Practices to Overcome Anxiety and Stress* by Regine Galanti

❖ *I Would, But My DAMN MIND Won't Let Me! A Teen's Guide to Controlling Their Thoughts and Feelings* by Jacqui Letran

❖ *My Anxious Mind: A Teen's Guide to Managing Anxiety and Panic* by Michael A. Tompkins and Katherine A. Martinez

❖ *Stuff That Sucks: A Teen's Guide to Accepting What You Can't Change and Committing to What You Can* by Ben Sedley

❖ *The Anxiety Survival Guide for Teens: CBT Skills to Overcome Fear, Worry, and Panic* by Jennifer Shannon and Doug Shannon

Creative Items to Help Reduce Anxiety for Kids

Since you've come this far, you know that no single antianxiety tool is going to do it all. Some kids enjoy more tactile, touch-based outlets while others may be soothed through creativity, connection, or relaxation. Here we give you a variety of ideas that your kids may enjoy.

❖ Kinetic sand/sand trays/sand tables

❖ Clay

❖ Squeeze balls

❖ Fidget toys (fidget cubes, fidget spinners, Rubik's Cubes, Tangle toys)

- ❖ Paint (finger painting or with brushes)
- ❖ Mandalas (Mandala is the Sanskrit word for magic circle and is a Hindu and Buddhist symbol representing the universe. Mandalas are considered a centering tool and have been used for centuries to evoke healing.)
- ❖ *Kids Basic Mandala Coloring Book* by Color Your World
- ❖ *Mandala Coloring Books for Kids: Zen Doodle* by Bowe Packer
  - ▸ *Kids' Magical Mandalas* by Arena Verlag
  - ▸ *Kids' First Mandalas* by Arena Verlag
  - ▸ *Preschool Mandala* by Blue Mountain
- ❖ Games
  - ▸ Stop, Relax, Think
  - ▸ The Talking, Feeling, and Doing Game
  - ▸ Go Fish: Anchor Your Stress
  - ▸ About Faces
  - ▸ My Calm Place

App and Website Resources to Help Reduce Anxiety for Kids

Use an online search engine or your phone's app store to find and explore these apps or to locate other options.

- ❖ Breathe, Think, Do Sesame
- ❖ Breathing Bubbles
- ❖ Calm
- ❖ Calm Counter
- ❖ Dreamy Kid

- ❖ Headspace

- ❖ Positive Penguins

- ❖ Smiling Mind

- ❖ Stop, Breathe, and Think Kids

- ❖ Take a Chill

Additional Kid-Friendly Antianxiety Resources

Use an online search engine to find and learn more about these interventions.

- ❖ ASMR for kids—ASMR (autonomous sensory meridian response) is a tingling sensation that begins on the scalp and moves down the neck and into the spine. It is considered very pleasant and mildly euphoric. The sensation, felt mostly on the arms and legs by those who experience it, can be triggered by certain sounds or images. Thousands of videos intended to stimulate ASMR have been posted on YouTube. Because YouTube also contains so much adult content, we highly recommend adult supervision for younger children or accessing videos through the YouTube Kids app.

- ❖ Mightier: Biofeedback Games for Kids—Biofeedback is a technique used to gain better awareness of the body's physiological functions, such as heart rate, in an effort to gain more control over it. By using electrical sensors, people receive feedback that allows them to make changes like relaxing muscles to calm themselves. This particular program uses your child's heart rate while playing video games to learn calming skills.

- ❖ GoZen!—This online stress management program offers educational videos and tools for parents, practitioners, and anxious kids to teach kids the science behind their anxiety as well as to help them develop coping skills.

Organizations and Websites with Additional Information about Anxiety

❖ Anxiety and Depression Association of America: https://adaa.org/

❖ AT Parenting Survival: https://www.anxioustoddlers.com

❖ The Child Anxiety Network: http://www.childanxiety.net/

❖ Child Mind Institute: https://childmind.org/

❖ National Alliance on Mental Illness: https://www.nami.org/

❖ Social Anxiety Association: http://socialphobia.org/

❖ Social Anxiety Institute: https://socialanxietyinstitute.org/

KYST Resources for Parents

We hope that one of the main things you take from this book is how important it is for caregivers and parents to take care of themselves. It is very difficult to KYST (see p. 33) when you are exhausted, overwhelmed, isolated, afraid . . . okay, you get the point. So we're not leaving adults out when it comes to resources. You'll find some more KYST ideas in the following lists.

Creative Items and Outlets to Help Reduce Anxiety for Parents

We already know you are doing so much to support your child (you bought this book!), but we want to make sure you are also taking care of yourself. It's so easy to minimize the need for emotional self-care, and we want to remind you that it is necessary for your well-being. You also can't do your best nurturing of others if you're not feeling emotionally well. Below we offer some ideas for how to channel your inner creativity and engage in helpful physical activities to make sure you are feeling your best.

❖ Color mandalas (see p. 154)

❖ Paint

❖ Play music

❖ Write

❖ Spend time with pets or animals

❖ Exercise

❖ Spend time with friends

❖ Spend time alone

❖ Journal

❖ Take a long bath

❖ Listen to your favorite podcast

❖ Call loved ones

❖ Clean/organize (only if it relaxes you!)

❖ Watch a funny movie

❖ Do yoga

App and Website Resources to Help Reduce Anxiety for Parents

Technology makes relaxation just a little bit easier. These applications offer meditations, guided imagery recordings, and sleep stories. Use an online search engine or your phone's app store to find and explore these apps or to locate similar options.

❖ Breathe2Relax

❖ Calm

❖ Happify

❖ Headspace

❖ Pacifica

❖ Rootd

❖ Tara Brach

Alternative Antianxiety Options for Parents to Try

We know that sometimes when people hear the term "self-care" they picture a spa retreat or a long run, but there are many ways for people to ease their anxiety. The following are not always the most top of mind or well-known outlets, but we know they have all been reported to reduce anxiety for some people. We also know that reducing anxiety is not one-size-fits-all, so it may be worth doing some investigating to see if one of these could be of interest to you.

❖ Acupuncture

❖ ASMR (autonomous sensory meridian response, found on various YouTube channels; see p. 155)

❖ Craniosacral therapy

❖ Cupping

❖ Essential oils

❖ Float therapy

❖ Massage

❖ Reiki

Build-Your-Village Resources for Parents

When it comes to resources we wanted to offer one additional thought: find your village. Raising kids is hard! Raising an anxious child comes with its own set of challenges, but you are not alone. One of the best KYST resources we can offer is to connect with other parents, share your challenges and your joys, laugh together, and cry together. Use an online search engine to find and explore these websites and blogs.

❖ AT Parenting Survival

❖ Hey Sigmund

- ❖ *Huffington Post* Parenting
- ❖ *New York Times* Parenting
- ❖ *Washington Post* On Parenting
- ❖ PEP Parent Encouragement Program
- ❖ Scary Mommy
- ❖ Therapy for Black Girls

Appendix

Understanding Anxiety-Related Structures and Processes

Understanding how anxiety manifests in the brain and the nervous system is complicated. Although this is not a comprehensive explanation of the complex processes that take place, we do want to provide a quick primer on the basics. For additional information, see the books listed on page 156.

Anxiety-Related Structures and Processes in the Brain and Nervous System

Limbic system: A complex set of structures within the brain that include the hippocampus, amygdala, hypothalamus, and thalamus. This is the area of your brain where emotional responses reside. It has influence over motivation, learning, and memory. It is also known as the "old brain"—the first area of the brain to develop in the human species.

Amygdala: A brain structure within the limbic system. This is where fear resides within the brain. It is also the brain structure that helps to prepare your body to react when there is an emergency. The amygdala is home to flight, fight, or freeze responses; it plays an important role in how anxiety manifests.

Hypothalamus: This brain structure helps keep things in the body balanced. It plays a role in many processes, including sleep cycles, body temperature, appetite, and emotions. The hypothalamus activates the sympathetic nervous system when the amygdala detects a threat, allowing your brain to tell your body to stay and defend yourself (fight), run away as fast as you can (flight), or not move a muscle (freeze).

Hippocampus: A structure within the limbic system that is important for the formation of new memories, solidification of memory, and navigating complex environments. The hippocampus is also related to emotion. Additionally, the hippocampus helps to activate the autonomic nervous system, which controls basic bodily functions.

Autonomic nervous system: This part of the nervous system is the "control center." It manages our basic bodily functions such as heartbeat, breathing, and digestion. It is a key player in our body's reactions to stress and anxiety. It is our physical nervous system reactions that tell our brain the story of why we are anxious. This area includes the sympathetic nervous system, which activates the fight, flight, or freeze reaction, and the parasympathetic nervous system, which helps the body relax after performing essential functions.

Prefrontal cortex: This is the structure in the brain that is responsible for planning, making decisions, and social behavior. It is part of the "new brain," which developed later in the evolutionary process in order to help people navigate our complex social world. This structure of the brain is the last one to develop as a person ages, continuing to grow and change until we are in our mid-twenties.

Neurotransmitters: Think of these as chemical messengers. When nerve cells want to communicate with each other, neurotransmitters are sent from a nerve cell to another nerve, muscle, organ, or tissue. These chemicals provide information to the cells. Dopamine, serotonin, histamine, and norepinephrine are all examples of neurotransmitters.

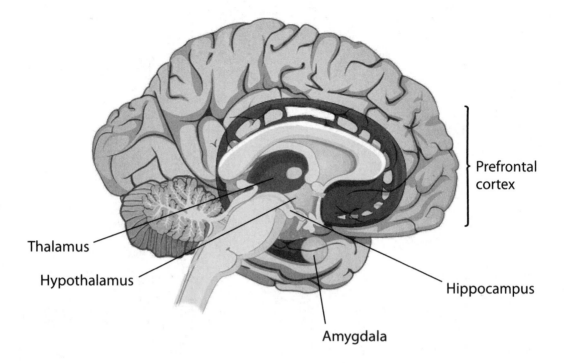

Thalamus

Hypothalamus

Prefrontal cortex

Hippocampus

Amygdala

Fight, flight, or freeze reaction: This is not a brain area but an important coping mechanism that allows our bodies to react as quickly as possible in dangerous situations (or situations that are perceived as dangerous). When faced with a threatening stimuli, the amygdala sends a signal to the hypothalamus, which activates the sympathetic nervous system. When this happens, the body releases hormones that provide energy to muscles and jump-start other bodily functions necessary to gather strength to fight off something dangerous, run as fast as possible away from it, or freeze in an attempt to be invisible to the threat (some predators' sight is based on movement). This reaction occurs automatically—before you are consciously aware that a threat is even present.

Appendix

Additional Support and
Professional Treatment Options

This book is designed to help you support your child. However, sometimes the interventions you put in place may not be enough. The number one piece of advice we have when it comes to intervention and support is that if you are unsure about what to do, *seek out a professional.* Your child may benefit from additional support or treatment. In this appendix, we address how you can go about finding that support.

And while we are at it, we want to mention that this information may be helpful for *you* too. If you feel that you may want to seek out additional support or treatment for yourself, the steps we outline on the next three pages are also applicable to finding personal help.

If you are . . .	Consider . . .	Which professionals can help you with this?	Other details to consider . . .
Just beginning to explore your concerns and decide what, if any, next steps are needed	An informal consultation	Pediatrician Primary care physician* School psychologist School counselor School social worker * If you have a close and comfortable relationship with a different type of medical provider, start there.	Speak to a professional you already know and/or is easily accessible to you. Schedule a quick meeting or call or catch them when they have a few minutes to talk privately.
Wanting to talk with a professional at length or have a thorough evaluation	A consultation with a mental health professional	Psychologist Social worker Licensed marriage and family therapist Licensed professional counselor	Ask a friend, other health service provider, or school staff if they have recommendations. Try an online search.[†] Contact your health insurance company and ask for recommendations in your network.[††] Contact the psychology or psychiatry department of a local college, university, or hospital.

See all footnotes on page 179.

Seeking a detailed evaluation that can identify mental health diagnoses and/or assess for developmental delays and learning disabilities by using standardized assessments	A neuropsychologist or psycho-educational evaluation	Clinical psychologist School psychologist	
Looking to: ■ Work through anxious thoughts and feelings ■ Gain further awareness and understanding for why these thoughts and feelings are there ■ Have more support and assistance with interventions	Beginning regular outpatient therapy sessions with a mental health professional[†††]	For your child, you may want to consider professionals with training in these types of therapy modalities: ■ Cognitive-behavioral therapy ■ Mindfulness-based therapy ■ SPACE (Supportive Parenting for Anxious Childhood Emotions) ■ Play therapy ■ Filial play therapy ■ Occupational therapy For yourself, there are so many different types of modalities and providers available that often it's just a matter of personal preference. Here we list a few that tend to be beneficial in the treatment of anxiety: (*continues on page 168*)	Definitely look for a professional who has expertise in anxiety as well as specific training to work with children. (If it's for you, they don't need the child expertise.) Depending on the age of your child, parent involvement may be a part of the process when you have a child in therapy. Some clinicians will meet with parents for full sessions; others will periodically touch base.

If you are . . .	Consider . . .	Which professionals can help you with this?	Other details to consider . . .
		▪ Acceptance and Commitment therapy ▪ Cognitive-behavioral therapy ▪ Dialectical-behavioral therapy ▪ Family systems ▪ Internal family systems ▪ Interpersonal therapy ▪ Mindfulness-based therapy ▪ Psychodynamic psychology	
Looking for more guidance and support on how to support your child in their anxiety	A parent consultation	Psychologist Social worker Licensed marriage and family therapist Licensed professional counselor	Many therapists offer this as a stand-alone option, or it can be included during the course of your child's therapy.
Looking to talk to someone about the risks and benefits of medication††††	A medication evaluation	Pediatrician (although some pediatricians will offer this, many do not) Psychiatrist Nurse practitioner Physician's assistant	A therapist may recommend that you consider medications, but only someone with a medical background can prescribe.

† If you are interested in doing an online search, here are some good starting points:

❖ PsychologyToday.com is a great search engine that allows you to target geographic locations and specific areas of specialty (e.g., children and anxiety).

❖ GoodTherapy.com

❖ TherapyForBlackGirls.com

❖ TherapyTribe.com

❖ Google "therapist" and your zip code

†† Some employers offer an Employment Assistance Program (EAP), which allows a certain number of visits with a licensed clinician (at no charge to the individual). These clinicians can typically only see the employee and not family members, but they may be a good starting point if you want to talk to someone about a longer-term plan.

††† Outpatient therapy does not have to be lengthy! It can be as short as eight weeks or as long as a person needs. (There is usually parental involvement in therapy for children.)

†††† Note that antidepressants are most often the preferred medical treatment for children. Medications are most likely to be used in conjunction with therapy.

Notes

Chapter 1

1. American Psychology Association, https://www.apa.org.
2. "What Are Anxiety Disorders?", American Psychiatric Association, https://www.psychiatry.org/patients-families/anxiety-disorders/what-are-anxiety-disorders.
3. "Anxiety Fact Sheet," American Academy of Pediatrics, https://www.aap.org/en-us/advocacy-and-policy/aap-health-initiatives/resilience/Pages/Anxiety-Fact-Sheet.aspx.
4. Ibid.
5. Kate Julian, "What Happened to American Childhood?" *The Atlantic*, May 2020, retrieved May 22, 2020, https://www.theatlantic.com/magazine/archive/2020/05/childhood-in-an-anxious-age/609079/.
6. "Any Anxiety Disorder," National Institute of Mental Health, https://www.nimh.nih.gov/health/statistics/any-anxiety-disorder.shtml.
7. Julian, "What Happened to American Childhood?"
8. Ibid.
9. Ibid.
10. "Facts and Statistics," Anxiety and Depression Association of American, https://adaa.org/about-adaa/press-room/facts-statistics.
11. Colleen M. Cummings, Nicole E. Caporino, and Philip C. Kendall. "Comorbidity of Anxiety and Depression in Children and Adolescents: 2 Years After," *Psychological Bulletin* 140, no. 3(May 2014), 816–845: https://doi.org/10.1037/a0034733.
12. David Beck Schatz and Anthony L. Rostain, "ADHD with Comorbid Anxiety: A Review of the Current Literature," *Journal of Attention Disorders* 10, no. 2, (November 1, 2006): 141–149. https://doi.org/10.1177/1087054706286698.
13. American Academy of Pediatrics, "Anxiety Fact Sheet."
14. Ibid.

Chapter 2

1. Gail Matthews, "Study Backs Up Strategies for Achieving Goals," Dominican University of California, 2011, http://www.goalband.co.uk/uploads /1/0/6/5/10653372/strategies_for_achieving_goals_gail_matthews_dominican _university_of_california.pdf.

Chapter 3

1. Stefan Koelsch et al., "Effects of Music Listening on Cortisol Levels and Propofol Consumption during Spinal Anesthesia," *Frontiers in Psychology* 2, no. 5 (2011), doi:10.3389/fpsyg.2011.00058; Elizabeth Landau, "This Is Your Brain on Music," CNN Health, January 23, 2018, https://www.cnn.com/2013/04/15/health/brain -music-research/index.html.
2. Colleen Vanderlinden, "It's True—You Really Should Talk to Your Plants," The Spruce, July 6, 2020, https://www.thespruce.com/should-you-talk-to -your-plants-3972298.

Chapter 4

1. Tarik Al-Kubaisy et al., "Role of Exposure Homework in Phobia Reduction: A Controlled Study," *Behavior Therapy* 23, no. (Autumn 1992): 599–621; Jennifer L. Podell and P. Kendall, "Mothers and Fathers in Family Cognitive-Behavioral Therapy for Anxious Youth," *Journal of Child and Family Studies* 20, no. 2 (2011):182–195.

Index

Page numbers followed by *t* indicate a table on the designated page

Notes

Notes

Notes

Notes

Notes

Notes

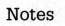
Notes